The Health House

1st Edition

The idea for this book has com[e as a result] of the books that I have read o[ver the years,] thought were relevant, I have listed in the appendix at the end of this book.

The book follows a simple principle that if you spent as much time dedicating yourself to the development of you as you do your house, then you would probably be in superb shape.

In fact, we take such good care of our houses that we insure them in case anything should happen to them. We have spent thousands of pounds and endless amounts of hours cleaning and improving them with such care and attention, only to leave them to our loved ones.

We spring-clean them each year, getting rid of all the clutter, and yet, we can carry things around in our heads for decades.

If life is always getting in the way, and you find yourselves making excuses as to why you are unhappy, self-conscious, anxious, unhealthy, then this is the time to digest the information in this book because it has been written with sole intention to help people make better choices in their lives.

'You are where you are in your life right now, as a result of the daily choices that you have made over the years.' ~ Tim Coates

We are genuinely excited for you because we know what a difference that the process in this book can make to you. We live and breathe this every day, and it only works!

Welcome to the only book that you will ever need to live the life, have the body and obtain the happiness that you desire.

Introduction & foreword 4
Results 11
Beliefs 22
What's Your Story 23
What's Your Strategy 29
Mind Your Language 32
Your potential 37
Thoughts 43
Some Science For You 48
A Bit More Science 52
Choices 57
Mind 68
Exercise 77
Nutrition 86
Sleep 94
Lifestyle 100
Detox your life 113
Dreams 118
Workbook 128
References and further reading: 165
Appendix 167

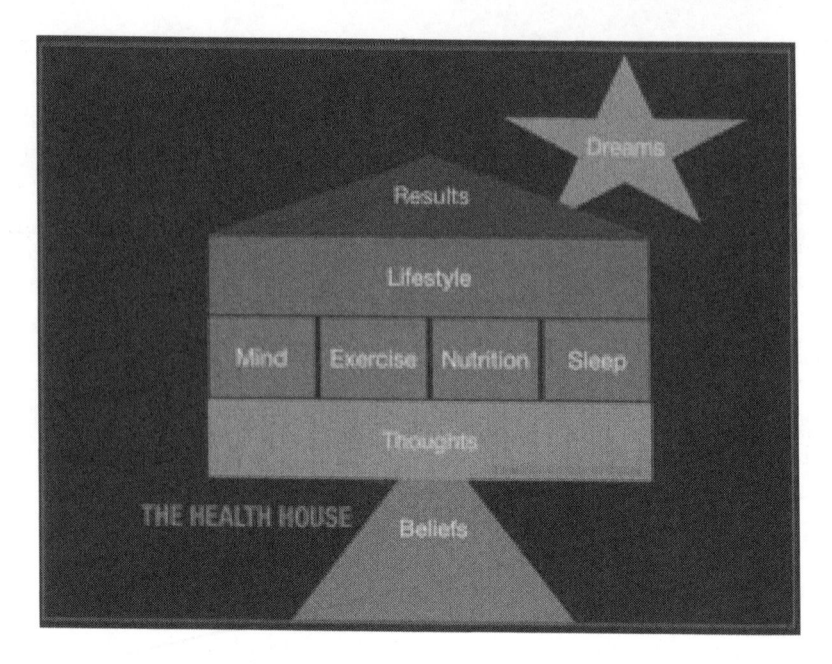

[Diagram: THE HEALTH HOUSE — showing a house shape with foundation "Beliefs", base "Thoughts", pillars "Mind", "Exercise", "Nutrition", "Sleep", roof section "Lifestyle", roof "Results", and a star labelled "Dreams" above.]

Introduction & foreword

I started this latest journey for several reasons actually, but I thought that I would share my thoughts and learnings along the way.

At 45 years old, I was somewhat overweight; even though I regularly exercised, it seemed that age and a diminishing metabolism had finally caught up with me.

I had an old knee injury that had prevented me from running for a few years and I had spent the previous year trying to fix it. My GP had told me that I should realise that it's part of getting old and I should just accept it.

I remember phoning my brother Damien from the car park feeling like I had been kicked in the stomach. He set me on a challenge to get into the very best shape that I could, just to prove the GP wrong.

Damien's approach is that you don't need to run for hours to lose weight and become healthier and providing I was willing to eat cleanly and commit to an exercise program, he would help me all he could.

Reason number two was that my wife and I had become a little comfortable in our own skins and had enjoyed life. As with everything, it catches up with you in the end. There is always that one photograph that someone takes of you, and when it is put on social media, you can hardly recognise yourself.

My photo was at a Christmas dinner with all my wife's family, and I looked like I had eaten myself. I didn't recognise myself at all. That was a catalyst for me as I had always been in a good athletic shape until now.

The third reason, and probably the most important, was that I wanted to inspire my wife to get healthy with me so that we can extend the amount of time that we have left with each other before the inevitable happens.

You see my wife's stepfather passed away after only a short battle with cancer, which crippled us all and hit me more than I could have anticipated. He and I had become close friends over the 20+ years that we knew each other, so I couldn't begin to imagine how my wife and her family felt.

Shortly after his passing, my wife became increasingly ill. We had been down the conventional route of seeing the GP, being referred to the hospital and having several false diagnoses. We finally decided to go private.

You see, there was a massive growth protruding through the stomach muscles, the size of which the specialist said they had never seen before. After a major operation and being bed bound for 3 months, I wanted my wife to make some changes and start a new healthy life after the warning that we had received.

On a positive note, we are all very healthy and we have already seen a huge change in our mindset, how and what we eat and our body shape after also going through regular exercise. We have been using all the tools and techniques in this book, and our hope is that you will also find the contents very useful.

So why a *Health* house? Well, I'm not a builder by any stretch of the imagination, but I have an understanding of how a house is built. I mean it has to have good foundations, quality bricks and mortar, water tight roof, etc. Most people will have lived in one at some point in their lives and will, therefore, be able to relate to how the book is structured.

The book starts with the *Results* roof because it is where everything in life appears to commence from these days. I mean we reduce everything into small bite-sized chunks of information, and we expect everything in an instant. We have become impatient because everything is available via the internet and the TV and we received constant streams of information on our smartphones at the touch of a button.

This book will explain why your continual obsession with your weight will only serve to demotivate you and that your outcome will depend on what you choose to focus your energy on. The following chapters will give details on how to stay focused and motivated to ensure that you achieve the shape that you want in your life. Like having a flat, pitched, glass or domed roof that, unless it is water tight, can be open to the elements and become warped.

Water is the one element that will always find the weakest point of the roof and begin the rotting process. Like water, if you allow yourself to be influenced by your external environment, you will consistently make bad choices.

Then we go to the very foundations of our house and, in particular, how we think, although I have referred this section to a pathway leading to the door of your mind. The importance of your beliefs and how they can affect your thoughts, behaviours and ultimately the results you achieve.

The human thought process is not as complex as you may think, and I have simplified it for everyone. I was taught a long time ago that if you can't explain it to your grandma, then you are over complicating it. The do's and don'ts of thinking for success, plus how you can take back control of your thoughts and how to make them work for you.

Choices are like the mortar between the building bricks of life that they can either hold everything together or cause things to come crashing down around us. The mistake that most people make is not realising that there is always a choice. You may not like the choice, but there is always one to be had and it is yours alone.

The building blocks of *Mindset, Exercise, Nutrition and Sleep* are directly influenced by your thoughts and choices that you make on a daily basis. You might be even making them at a subconscious level without even realising. Hopefully, this book will go some way to showing you how to take control back.

What is life without a dream? Dr Martin Luther King said, 'I have a dream,' and it started a movement with regards to the civil rights of black people in America. It wouldn't have been the same if he'd said, 'I have a goal,' would it? It is in our DNA as human beings to dream of things we aspire to because if we can dream it, then we can achieve it.

Most innovative inventions have come from the question, 'Wouldn't it be good if...' Virgin Atlantic was born from the need of Richard Branson to charter an aircraft from Los Angeles. It is okay to dream because it allows us to fulfil those basic human needs to constantly evolve – without imagination, we would still be living in caves.

In the second part of the book, you will find a 30-day-detox-your-mind program, with a daily task and thought-provoking questions that I would use if I were coaching you 1-2-1.

Carefully read through the daily task and complete everything in order. If you miss a day, just start from where you left off. You will need to complete the whole program which will include weekends. It doesn't mean that you only do this Monday to Friday but it does mean that you NEED to complete 30 consecutive days in a row.

Why should you detox your brain? Well, if you have ever wondered why most diets and fitness programs fail, then you will understand what I am about to say. Before you embark on any fitness or eating plan, you must first prepare your mind to make the necessary sacrifices. Get your mindset right first, and everything else will fall into place; get it wrong, and it is like building a house on uneven foundations.

You will find links to our online community as well as useful templates throughout the book but particularly in the appendix. Let's get started because it's time to spring-clean your mind.

Acknowledgements

I would like to dedicate this book to my wife for always putting up with me working long hours and my incessant need for her love and unconditional support.

My son, Christopher, for always believing in me and encouraging me with his kind words.

To Chester (my dog) for the way he greets me and for making me feel like a rockstar when I come home.

My parents, Ray and Janice Coates, for the life experiences and support that they have given me over the last 45 years.

To my baby brother, Damien Coates, and his fiancée, Lianne Sykes, for getting me involved in their fitness business and for their continued support and hard work.

To my older brother, Lee Coates, his wife, Sarah, and their two children, Lewis and Lacey, thanks for the advice and the country walks with the dogs.

To all my friends and family who have encouraged me, supported me and cared for me over the years. I am extremely grateful to you all.

Foreword & testimonials

Everyday life can get overwhelmingly busy without you realising, this course helped me to switch off from that and reconnect with myself. The exercises are a great way to open your mind and appreciate the good in every moment. - Kerry Weldon

My mindset has never been better! Better than a course of CBT. - Nicola Howarth

Following the 30 day mind & body detox program Tim guided us through how our minds have the power to adapt to changes in a positive way through a series of tasks. He showed us how having a positive mindset can change your outlook on life and help you achieve the things you never believed you could. The program helped me achieve my goal & changed how I view my life. - Kayte Smyth

A really powerful approach that addresses all aspects of your life in order to succeed. It provided me with an easy to follow and realistic set of mind tools to help me achieve my goals, and manage my challenges successfully. As a health care professional the principles in the book are so pertinent are to all medical staff and patients. In the ever changing and challenging NHS landscape we need these tools to survive, thrive and take care of ourselves. - Many Giblin

Chapter 1
Results

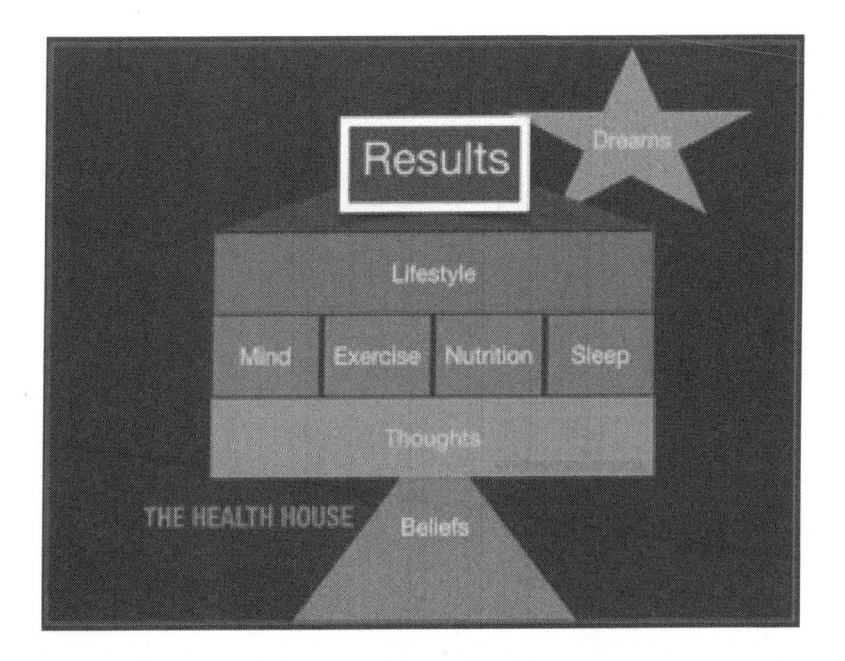

We are constantly bombarded with the latest FITNESS CRAZES and FADS that promise UNBELIEVABLE results, at what price?

If you ARE happy, then continue with whatever you are doing because you clearly have this sewn up; if not, then you will want to continue reading.

'The definition of madness is to consistently do the same thing over and over again AND expect a different result' ~ Albert Einstein.
Here is a simple fact: if you are not getting the results that you want, then you NEED to do something different!

We are so fixated on results that we can often forget the PRICE that we need to pay to get whatever it is that we have set our hearts upon. We reduce everything to simple statistics from our bodies, business, sport and even poetry, for goodness sake.

As meter and rhyme is a way to measure poetry, sports matches are reduced to scores, successful passes, fouls committed, etc. The emotion and passion are therefore lost in the translation, much like reducing the human form down to weight, measurements, BMI and fat percentages.

There are no shortcuts to a good body shape or healthy lifestyle because the price is still the price. You can't ask LIFE for a discount on that price or demand that TIME gives you a 25% reduction. That is like trying to put a roof on your house when you haven't built the walls yet – it's ridiculous, right?

In my experience, results come down to the following equation:

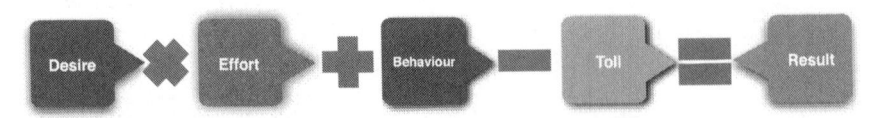

$$\text{Desire} \times \text{Effort} + \text{Behaviour} - \text{Toll} = \text{Result}$$

If your DESIRE is greater than the TOLL, then you will always manage to find the EFFORT and energy needed to achieve the RESULT you want. That is providing that you are to able to commit to habitual BEHAVIOUR and resilience to keep you on that track. We will discuss it more in the next chapter.

The Toll that I paid is countless early mornings and hours in the gym, the money spent on the right nutrition and supplements each month; the time away from my friends and family and the strict daily disciplines that meant no caffeine, alcohol, treats and other favourite foods.

If you are STILL NOT getting the results that you want AND you always seem to catch yourself saying the same things, then ask yourself, 'Do I want it badly enough, or is the price simply too high?'

If you do, then we will show you how to overcome ANY barrier that life can throw at you AND how to become happier in the process.

In today's society, we have a knack of reducing everything to a number or statistic, which is not always the best scenario when dealing with the emotions of desire.

When it comes to the affairs of the heart, sometimes our choices are illogical and defy the laws of statistics. For example, have you ever watched a sports game on your television and spent the whole game shouting at the TV?

Most of us have, but why do we do it? We know that there is nothing that we can do to affect the game or the referee's decision, and yet we get so caught up in the passion of the game. Reality completely eludes us, which is ridiculous considering we could be hundreds of miles away from the stadium.

Some of my clients have been professional sportsmen and women over the years, and some of the cars that they have turned up in are stunning. Like most men, I have an affinity for beautiful cars and so I take an interest, and they freely answer all my questions due to the level of rapport that we have.

'What made you choose that particular car, colour, model, etc.,' I often ask because I want to know where their thoughts were when they made that particular choice. Often they will just reply, 'I just liked it,' and that is precisely what I mean when I say that emotional desire can often hold no logic.

You see, if the car has cost the best part of £100k and has a rocketing depreciation value, logic would say that they would be better off choosing a mainstream, although less luxurious, brand. If you are an accountant, you might not make such rational decisions.

For the record, I love beautiful cars and would buy one in a heartbeat because life is too short not to indulge once in a while.

The point I am making is that as much as we try to reduce everything to statistics, it is not what being human is all about.

There is a film called *The Prisoner* (1967) and it is about a retired secret agent who is abducted and taken to what appears to be an idyllic village only to discover that it is a prison. The wardens demand information from him, but he endeavours to escape, and he is only ever referred to by his prison number, which is 6.

In what has now become an iconic scene, during an interrogation, he shouts, 'I am not a number, I am a free man.'

What is really amusing is that we reduce ourselves to numbers too.

We seem obsessed by how much we weigh, and I was just as guilty as the next person. For example, during my 'building muscle' phase, I was always checking my weight after each workout. I just wanted to see if I had put on any more mass, only to feel constantly disappointed.

The same could be said for my wife on the lead up to our wedding. She was consistently checking to see if she had lost any more weight overnight.

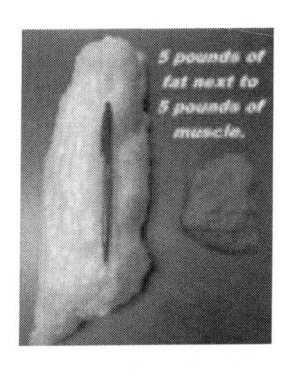

The point that I need to make very clear is that in the photo opposite lie 5lbs of fat and 5lbs of muscle. As you can see muscle is far smaller than fat, and yet they both weigh the same.

This means that as you exercise, your muscles become denser, which signifies that you might lose dress sizes but still weigh the same.

We have re-named the scales in our house as the 'sad steps'. This is because we don't know anyone who is ever happier when they step off the scales. Whether you are trying to put weight on or lose weight, you will never be satisfied with your result.

If you are an athlete or a body builder that is competing in a particular category, then I can understand the need for strict and almost obsessive weight loss/gain. How many of you that are reading this book will be competing, though? If you are, you should contact us at info@theleanbodyproject.com, and we will put you in touch with one of our Professional PTs.

Instead of focusing on your weight, focus on your shape! That way you will notice that your clothes become loose and your stomach looks flat in that dress that you bought for the Christmas party, etc.

By all means, take photographs of your journey because it will spur you on when you can see your body transforming in front of your eyes. It will also be an excellent way to celebrate your success and relive the journey once you hit your target shape.

Make a note of all your measurements too because you might not notice a change in the mirror from week to week, although you may see that your arms or your thighs are getting smaller and that your clothes are looser, and that will encourage you to continue.

There WILL come a time throughout the journey when you will want to throw in the towel. When the place where you started before your transformation suddenly becomes more desirable than your destination. It is at this point you will need a good group of like-minded people or community around you to keep you going.

'As long as you are pointing the right direction, then keep moving, and you will get there eventually.' ~ Buddha

Also, from our most famous leader, Winston Churchill, comes the quote: 'If you are going through hell, keep going.' Meaning that in the end, you will come out on the other side. The important message is to keep moving, making progress no matter how small or seemingly insignificant.

There are so many nutritional plans and super fast exercise programs out there, and most have been celebrity endorsed too.

I have yet to find a single silver bullet that will work for everyone in the world because there are too many variables to contend with. What I mean by that is that what might work for your friend because she has seen amazing results doesn't mean that it will work for you too, and you will be disappointed when you won't get the same results.

It's back to that *Results* word again. Let's face it, we all want a particular outcome and we want to get it the most efficient and quickest way possible, right?

Regardless of the exercise and nutrition program, unless you have your mind set in the direction that you want to go, you will inevitably be led by your impulses (your subconscious mind) and more likely give in to your cravings.

The truth of the matter is that providing you have your mindset fixed on where you are going and have properly prepared it by detoxing your brain beforehand, then you will be more likely to make better choices when it comes to exercise and eating.

Mindset, exercise and nutrition are a trinity of equal importance and are the elements to your success. If any of these factors are missing or are weak, then the likelihood of you being successful diminishes significantly.

Only when you have a strong mindset, will you make the right choices on a daily basis about your nutrition and your exercise. It all starts in your mind first.

Imagine a three-legged stool for a second, similar to the one that a milkmaid might use to milk a cow. If one of those legs were weak, you could well imagine what would happen if the milk maid were to sit down on it every day. Eventually, it would collapse, and the milk maid would inevitably end up on the floor.

If per se, the stool only has two legs, then it is still usable providing the other two are sturdy enough to support her weight. It may be a little wobbly and unbalanced but useable nonetheless.

The similarities are there for us to acknowledge because if we have one weak element, it will be like losing a leg from the stool. Our commitment will become wobbly and unstable. When we have all three aspects present and each as strong as the others, then we are absolutely sure we will achieve our goals.

Top tip: Start by getting your mind geared up for what is coming first before you embark on an expensive commitment of joining a gym or signing up for personal training. Likewise, research the eating plans thoroughly and NEVER diet; instead, find a nutritional plan that works for you. We have several available via www.theleanbodyproject.com for you to have a play with.

As I said before, there is no 'one size fits all' when it comes to living a healthier life. Everyone is different: we all have different metabolisms, blood types, lifestyles, energy levels, ailments and hormone levels. Not everyone's lifestyle is the same, some people can handle stress better than others, sleep patterns vary from 2-10 hours per night, etc. I could go on, but you get the picture.

Your journey to becoming healthy or having the body that you want I believe is the most important aspect of this whole chapter.

First of all, it becomes a lifestyle choice for you – it is never a diet or a fad. How many people do you know that have lost loads of weight over a few months only to put it all back on, plus a few pounds extra?

It is the diet versus discipline effect. When people diet, they stick to a plan for a relatively short period of time and then once they get to their deadline, they turn right back. They do all of the undisciplined things that they did before that made them unhappy in the first place and pile all their weight back on again and more besides.

I remember one client, she was getting married within six months and she was desperate to get to a target size 12 from 16. We worked hard for almost five months leading up to the wedding, and she looked superb at a size 10.

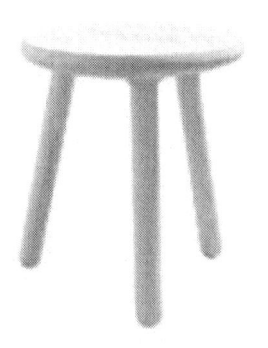

Rate yourself on a scale of 1-10 on how strong you are at the following areas:

Mindset: 1 - I crumble at the first temptation or 10 - I am so disciplined only a hurricane could deter me

Exercise: 1 - I never get involved in exercise or 10 - I exercise every day like a machine

Nutrition: 1 - Fast food is my best friend or 10 - I

Six months after her marriage, she came back to us to go through it all again. You see, she had gone back to her old habits and within 6 months she was back to square one, unhappy and back up to size 18.
Which areas of your life are you the strongest at and which parts do you need to work on?

Chances are, if you are reading this book, you are not yet getting the results that you want. The good news is that you CAN have those results that you are so determined to have, providing you re-think your targets.

According to researchers, they have found that the depiction of the ideal female body chosen by both men was fairly consistent with the women's choice and was based on:

- Body Mass Index (BMI) = mass kg/height m2
- Waist-to-hip Ratio (WHR) = Circumference of Waist/ Circumference of Hips

- Waist-to-chest Ratio (WCR) = Circumference of Waist/ Circumference of Chest

In an attempt to reduce the beauty of a female body to statistics, the emotion of desire has been lost in the translation. I mean I have never EVER seen a man weigh up a girl whose looks he likes and check her against this so-called 'chart of perfection'.

Instead, what happens is an emotional connection that is created between two human beings regardless of her or his measurements.

Some would have us believe that we have to count every calorie, sin or treat each day, weigh our food and check out every ingredient that is listed on the packet.

If you are like me, you think that life is busy enough and you just want something that you can stick to that will help you get into the shape you desire. Simples!

I want something really simple to understand and easy to stick to. Is that too much to ask?

We will cover my approach to nutrition and exercise in the later chapters but for now, let's keep this high level.

Cut out sugar from your diet completely! No need to weigh it, count it or save up your sins, just STOP using it. The latest evidence describes sugar as lethal as class-A drugs and just as addictive.

The one biggest thing that you can do to improve your health right now if you are overweight, you suffer from diabetes, heart complaints, headaches and high cholesterol is to cut sugar from your life once and for all.

Try it for 30 days and notice the difference. What have you got to lose?

The world's leading health experts have publicly announced that sugar is the new smoking, in that it has such a dramatic impact on our bodies. Premature ageing, dementia, Alzheimer's, diabetes and cancer are just a few of the diseases attributed to sugar.

Dr Aseem Malhotra is a world leading cardiologist and former clinical associate to the Academy of Medical Royal Colleges, and Dr Hyman is the Medical Director at Cleveland Clinic's Centre for Functional Medicine, the Founder of The UltraWellness Centre, and a ten-time #1 New York Times Best-selling author.

They are both leading the way to change our relationship with sugar and ultimately help us make better choices when it comes to the amount that we consume. Reduce the quantity a little at a time, so for example, if you take two spoonfuls of sugar in your tea or coffee, reduce it to one for a few days and then down to half, etc.

Summary

- Remember that your desire multiplied by your effort, plus your resilience, minus the price equates to the result that you will achieve. If you are not happy with the results you are getting, which one of these areas will you need to work on?

- Focus on the right set of results and bin the sad step! Concentrate on your measurements, from around your arms, waist and thighs. Take photos of your journey one side on and the other full frontal (in underwear or bikini).

- Remember that muscle weighs more than fat! The more you exercise, the more muscle mass you will acquire, and the type of exercise will determine the total amount. This is hugely beneficial for your health because, amongst other things, it helps to keep all your internal organs in place by strengthening your internal corset.

- Are all of your core elements in alignment with your goals? Does your mindset contribute to or take you away from your goal? You can have the very best nutrition and exercise program that money can buy but if your mindset isn't prepared, it will only work against you and you will hate every minute.

- Sugar is fast growing to be public enemy number one and, with more evidence becoming available each day, the single biggest change that you can make to your health is to cut out the sugar!

Chapter 2
Beliefs

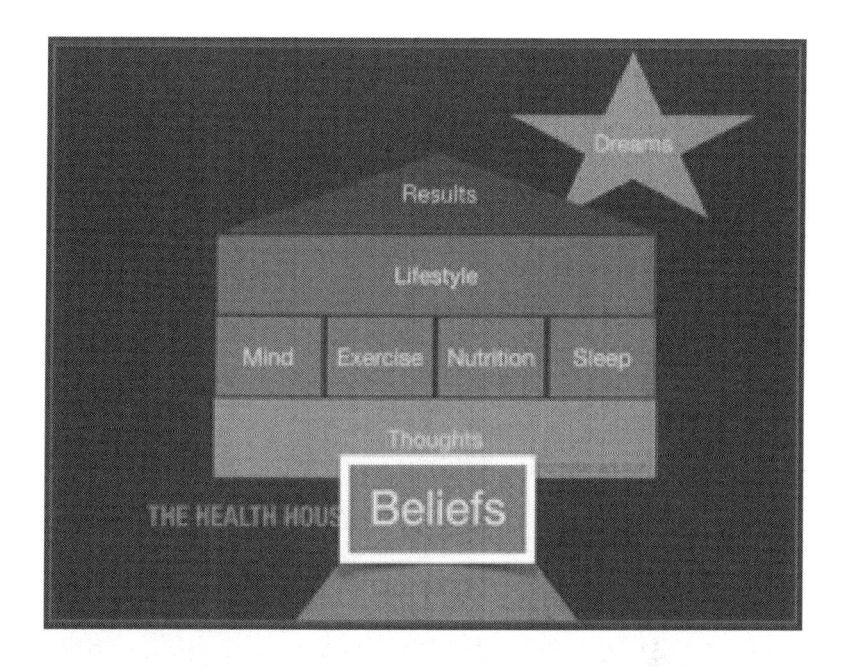

What's Your Story

If our BELIEFS are underpinned by our VALUES, where do we get our values from?

There is scientific evidence that we get our values from a number of places, including:
- Parents - we can adopt the examples and opinions from our parents
- Environment - it includes your friends, school, social scene, etc.
- Genetic Pre-Disposition - the hardwired neural network of the brain

If you are one of the lucky ones AND you are happy with everything in your life including how you look, then you are one in a million that are already doing what I am about to suggest.

'Your subconscious mind is eavesdropping on your thoughts and acting accordingly.' ~ Deepak Chopra.

Deepak Chopra is an American author, and his books include 'quantum healing' and 'super brain'. He developed a way of harnessing the power of your thoughts to heal your own body of its afflictions from the inside out.

The way that you THINK impacts upon what you believe, how you behave, how successful you are, how you feel, your confidence and ultimately your happiness.

Your THOUGHTS precede everything in your life, and you adjust yourself accordingly, mentally, physically and spiritually.

Change the way that you think and you change everything. Would you like to know the SECRET of how to make your thoughts work for you?

It starts with what you focus on AND the language that you use!

If you focus on all the things that you don't have, then you will never have them. If you come from a place of sincere GRATITUDE, then you are starting from a place that is both positive and powerful. Science argues that feeling grateful actually alters the neural networks in your brain AND affects how you FEEL.

By focusing on the things that you want in your life, rather than the things that you don't want, you are more likely to succeed in your ambitions, e.g. how many times have you heard someone say, 'I want to lose weight'? Probably a few, right? The very language suggests that the person is focusing on 'losing weight', which will have a negative impact on their thoughts and their success.

A more positive spin would be 'I want to become healthier'.

> THE STORY THAT YOU TELL YOURSELF IS JUST AS IMPORTANT AS YOUR STRATEGY.

Why does putting something into a positive statement matter so much?

We will explore the process of human thinking in the next chapter, although this will lay the foundations for us to comprehend just how impact our beliefs in the process.

You see the mind cannot differentiate between imagination and reality without our fundamental beliefs. These come from our experiences in life which are either good or bad.

Tony Robbins calls them 'SEE' (Significant Emotional Experiences), and they can define not only the story we tell the world but, first and foremost, the one we tell ourselves.

The year 2016 was a catalyst for me personally and definitely a SEE that could have completely devastated every aspect of my world.

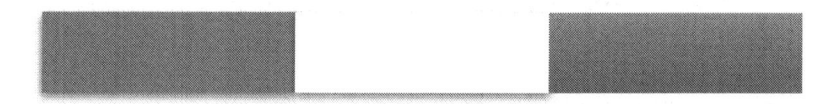

We lost a very dear friend in the September of the previous year, which left an enormous void in most of my families lives. My father-in-law was a large Italian gentleman who can best be described as a 'character' by some and a loveable rogue by others. It is very easy to underestimate the impact of loss on your own beliefs.

He had battled aggressive cancer from the January of that same year, and although it happened over 9 months, the treatments took their toll immediately. Still, he kept his spirits up, and we as a family were able to enjoy the last family holiday in his beloved Italy in August, one month before he passed. He died in the UK, just 7 days after his return.

He added joy into everybody's life that he knew and even through his most difficult days, he was able to model his beliefs. He believed that:

- A dinner table should be filled with family and friends.
- Good wine is made better when shared
- We should live to eat and NOT eat to live
- Good nutritious food should be tasty

You see all the specialists were telling him that he was too weak to travel to Italy and that we should make preparations for his passing whilst in Italy.

I sincerely believe that it was his sheer determination and self-belief that allowed him to have one last holiday with his family AND return safely, just as he predicted!

So what is your story? What is that you are telling yourself that is STOPPING you from committing to or achieving your goals?

The SEE of losing my father-in-law had a devastating impact on my wife and all her family, especially my mother-in-law. This, in turn, had a significant impact on my marriage, which had a huge personal toll.

The story that I began to tell myself was that travelling to Italy would never feel the same and I began to DREAD the thought of going back.

The reality was that we had purchased a house in a beautiful spot in the mountains, with the most amazing views of the vineyards and mountain ranges. It is truly breathtaking, and we are extremely fortunate to have been in such a position to make it our home.

We did return the following year and, if anything, it has made us more appreciative of the time that we spent there and filled us with excitement for the memories that we have yet to write there.

Things will happen in your life and may have already happened in your past that you STILL carry around with you today.

It is like holding a glass half-filled with water with your arm outstretched. You can hold this for at least 5 minutes and you should find it fairly easy. If you continue for an hour or two, it becomes quite uncomfortable and possibly painful. Now imagine holding that glass for 10, 20 or even 30+ years, it is going to feel really heavy, right?

If you were told that you were fat at school when you were 9 years old and you were bullied throughout your junior years, you might suffer from low self-esteem due to that SEE, but if you continue to tell yourself that you are still that 9 year old, then guess what? You are going to believe it!

Have you ever had anyone in your life tell you that you can't do something? I know that I have and, being the stubborn rebel that I can be, it often makes me more determined to prove those people wrong. I don't publicly declare my intentions but rather allow my actions to do the talking for me.

You see, if someone tells you that you are worthless or that you will never make anything of yourself consistently enough, you begin to believe it! If someone has been telling you that you are fat and ugly for a few years, then you start not only to believe it but also to ACCEPT it.

This is part of the belief cycle because once you have accepted the opinions of others as YOUR TRUTH, then you will also begin to self-fulfil that prophecy!
If you are still telling yourself that you are not worthy or that you don't deserve love and connection, then guess what? You will feel unhappy and very lonely too.

Take a moment to listen to some of the stories that you are telling yourself as to why you cannot:

A. Eat healthier
B. Commit to exercise
C. Stick to the plan

On each of these areas, grade yourself on a scale of 1-10, 1 being I don't do this at all to 10 being I do this every day without thinking.

Are you ready to put the glass of water down now?

Good. Because the story is only part of the jigsaw and as any good storyteller would say, 'It's the way you tell your story that matters, just as much as the story itself.'

> Your brain doesn't process negative language.

We have already mentioned the power of language, and its impact, both positive and negative alike. Now we are going to examine some of the words and language that you are using when you tell your story especially to yourself.

The language we choose to use on a daily basis will determine the results that we will achieve at the end of the day.

For example:
'I am too old now to do anything about my weight, my doctor has told me that I shouldn't do any vigorous exercise due to my bad knee.' or

'I exercise 4+ times per week and yet I still can't lose weight.'

If you are telling others that you are too old to work out, then you are reinforcing your own beliefs that you are too old to do anything. Also, who said that you need to do vigorous exercise to lose weight? There are also other types of workout that you can do that will have minimal impact on your knee. Just because you are unable to run for 30 minutes, doesn't mean that you couldn't eat healthier and reduce your alcohol intake.

If you are exercising four times or more a week and not losing weight, then it will suggest either that:

- You're not working hard enough
- You need to redesign your program because your body gets used to it after 6 weeks
- You are eating the wrong things and need to change what you are eating
- Or you have a physical deficiency (Thyroid) and should seek a medical opinion

You see, the language that is used on a daily basis becomes important, and we are surrounded by negative language all day, which affects us on a subconscious level without us even being aware of it.

How many of you put the news on first thing in the morning and leave it on whilst completing your pre-work routine? Tell me, is there ever anything positive on the news, or is it all doom and gloom?

Do you listen to a radio station in the car on the way to work? What does your preferred station tell you about your current mindset?

When you get into work, are you met with positivity each day or do you have any of those "fun sponges"? You know, they are these people that are all doom and gloom that suck all the positivity from everyone before moving on to their next victim.

The truth is we are subconsciously affected by all of those elements on a daily basis and we can recognise it most in our own language.

An old adage is that you will either find a way or find an excuse!

Write down your story overleaf. You know, that one that you have been telling yourself for a long time and be honest with yourself. Tip: If you are brave enough, ask someone that knows you very well to do this for you, just ask them to be sincere! Also, you must accept what they write without trying to defend yourself, remember that it will come from a place of love for you. Just say thank you!

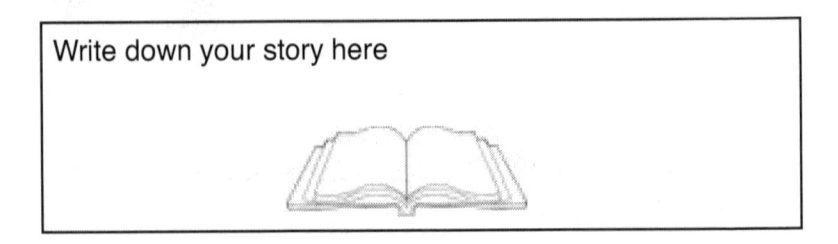

Write down your story here

What's Your Strategy

What is your strategy for getting the life that you want, or do you not have a plan yet?

More importantly, who do you need to become for you to have the life that you have dreamed of?

Most people will have you believe that to have something manifest itself in your life, you need to visualise that you already have it and feel it with all the fibres in your body. I'm not suggesting that this doesn't work, but that sometimes destiny could use a little effort from us too.

Coaching is very much a privilege, and I am truly humbled by the people that have allowed to share their personal and professional journey with them. To this day, I still work with a small selection of coaching clients but I choose to keep them to an intimate level now.

I haven't just told you this to impress you but rather impress upon you that some of the more ambitious of my clients first came to me frustrated that their strategy for promotion to the top table had passed them by.

This is because of a very simple principle in that those on the board haven't deemed them to be ready. This doesn't mean that they should leave the company, but instead find what area of personal development needs to take place for those few board members to approve their exclusive membership.

Ask yourself WHO do you need to become first for you to be ready when the opportunity arises?

Where can you find the knowledge that you need to better your understanding of that role in life?

The same stands when it comes to having a healthier life. What should you be reading? What seminars could you attend? Where are the lectures being held? Where do like-minded people hang out?

When I went to university, I quickly learned to spend time with the people in the year above me. WHY? Because they held the answers to what I was about to experience. It wasn't asking for their answers or plagiarism, it was simply getting ahead. You see, if you spend time with those that are more knowledgeable than you, then you are bound to pick things up.

There are soooo many diets, exercise plans, nutrition plans, and they all profess to be revolutionary, especially when it comes to losing weight and getting healthy.

As a former PT, I thought that I knew all that I needed to know about all things related to health and well-being, but I didn't take into account the loss of metabolism. Our metabolism slows down with age, and even with tremendous amounts of exercise, I still retained my middle-age spread.

So I spent countless hours debating with my brother, Damien Coates, a number one bestselling author on Amazon with The Lean Body Solution. We have done all the hard work so that you, the reader, don't have to, and we have collated it into this one book! The only book that you should ever need.

We wanted to simplify the whole process and ditch the hype and BS. Our aim is to focus the things that have been proven time and time again to help people lose weight and become healthier. We have read thousands upon thousands of books, attended numerous conferences and spent half a century in the industry.

We have researched people like Joe Wicks for his recipes, Aseem Malhotra the world's leading cardiology expert for nutritional advice and Tony Robbins for a little motivation. We have read countless books including Hal Elrod's 'Miracle Morning' and Darren Hardy's 'Compound Effect'. A full list is available in the appendix should you be interested.

In the words of the late Stephen Covey, 'Start with the end in mind' I also add the words of Hal Elrod, a wise philosopher, 'You are always exactly where you are supposed to be, experiencing what you need to experience in order to learn what you must learn to become the person that you need to be to create the life that you truly want.'

It is not enough to have the perfect plan in place, you must apply action to it, and before you even do that, you must first become that person who is able to execute that plan.

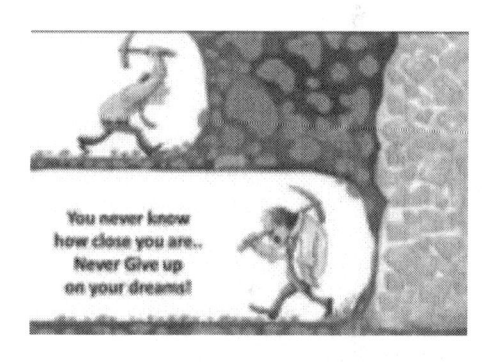

How much time do you spend daily reading or investing in yourself?

Now, looking at your day, how can you expect to develop yourself if you don't dedicate some time to develop your mind?

You could join the Facebook group online where you can chat with like-minded people that have either been where you are or are there now and want to share their journey with you. Free 30-day weight loss challenge

Mind Your Language

> Itemise your daily routines from the moment you wake to the moment you go to sleep:

We've already touched on language briefly, and I want to delve a little deeper right now.

If Deepak Chopra is indeed correct by saying that every cell in your body is eavesdropping on your thoughts, then understand this: Every thought that you have is listening to every word that you say both internally and externally.
If you have been told not to do something, what did you do?

Imagine that your subconscious mind reacts like a 4-year-old child when you say to it, 'Don't touch that wall it has just been painted.' What will it do?

Yep, you guessed it, they'll go and touch it.

It is the same when you say to that four-year-old carrying a cup of juice, 'Don't spill the juice.' Guess what will happen. Having experienced this first hand (Lacey May), they will concentrate on not spilling it that they will start to shake and ultimately spill it.

A much better way of saying this would have been: 'Please be very careful with that juice.' Same message, just different words.

Why does this matter so much? Well, the brain doesn't process the negative word in the sentence, 'DON'T', and hears the command of 'SPILL THE JUICE' instead.

When my clients tell me that they don't do healthy eating because either they don't have the time or it's too expensive, I often test their desire to get healthy. Opting for 'How serious are you?' Or 'What is more important to you, your health or saving a few pounds?'

When a child says, 'I can't,' as adults what do we say to them? 'There is no such thing as "can't".' Just that statement alone reinforces their belief that they can't. If you remove the negatives from the sentence, then you end up with 'there is such a thing as "can't".' An alternative way to say this may be to delete the T. If you ask the child to remove the 'T' from 'can't', what do you end up with? CAN.

How often do you tell yourself that you can't do something? I can't come to the gym tonight because... or I can't do any more push ups or I can't prepare clean meals in advance because I don't know what I might fancy, etc.

Delete the T because you can do all of those things as long as you tell yourself that you CAN. Henry Ford once said, 'Whether you believe you can or you can't, you are right.' In other words, whatever you tell yourself that you CAN do, you are more likely to achieve.

I just love this next word in a sentence: TRY. Whenever I hear that particular word, I know that the person is not going to do what I asked. Why? In the famous words of YODA, 'do or do not, there is no try.'

I was once invited to a street party in the UK to celebrate the royal wedding of Kate and William. My reply was 'I'll try and make it' which meant I wasn't going to go but I was too polite to just decline. I also want to clarify that I wasn't actually invited to THE Royal wedding, this was a street party in Manchester some 200 miles away. Otherwise, I'd have been there in a heartbeat.

When my clients say, 'I'll try,' I instinctively know that 9/10 times they are implying 'this ain't happening,' so I will move in for more of commitment from them.

When you can really listen to someone's words as well as the message, then you often read between the lines, which makes for a good coach.

Thanks to AncientWisdomTrail.com for creating the figure overleaf which nicely demonstrates in good detail the explanation of how language affects our whole being.

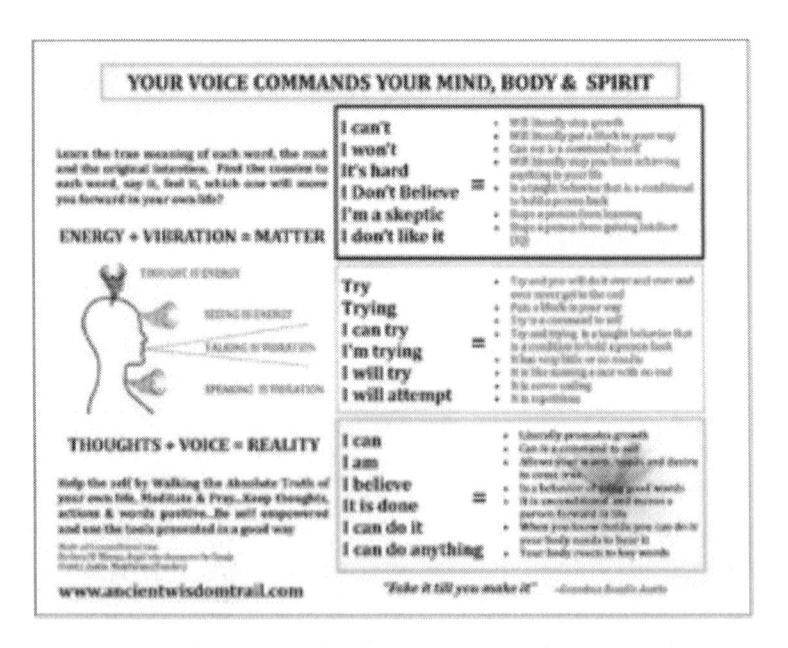

YOUR VOICE COMMANDS YOUR MIND, BODY & SPIRIT

ENERGY + VIBRATION = MATTER
- I can't
- I won't
- It's hard
- I Don't Believe
- I'm a skeptic
- I don't like it

THOUGHTS + VOICE = REALITY
- Try
- Trying
- I can try
- I'm trying
- I will try
- I will attempt

- I can
- I am
- I believe
- It is done
- I can do it
- I can do anything

www.ancientwisdomtrail.com

I was watching the Scottish Election one year, about the time when there was a scandal concerning the UK Ministers of Parliament regarding their expenses. One Scottish MP said, 'I'm not saying that all MPs are lying, cheating thieves,' which made me giggle. What they were saying is that 'all

English MPs were lying, cheating thieves.' Someone should have sensor-checked their speech beforehand.

Another example is the famous former President of the USA, Bill Clinton, 'I did not have sexual relations with that woman,' referring to the now famous Monica Lewinsky. What was he really saying?

Now that we have a little understanding of such language, HOW does this affect our thoughts?

Our brains have two separate hemispheres connected only by a neural pathway called the 'corpus callosum'. Your brain also has a conscious and a subconscious mind also. One allows you to focus and concentrate on detail when you need to but it has limited capacity, and the other deals with about 4 billion bits of information per second (I'd love to know how they calculated this number).

Whatever you say in your conscious mind when you are thinking or having a conversation has an impact on your subconscious mind also. I liken the conscious mind to your awake and adult mind, and the subconscious as your inner child like a 4-year-old.

You see, whatever your conscious mind (adult) says vocally or inside your head, your subconscious mind (child) believes it and delivers what you have just said to it. For example, I can't go to the gym because I've left my trainers at home. Your subconscious mind reinforces that, and you probably won't get to the gym.

Your language (positive or negative) impacts your thoughts, which in turn has an affect on your choices that ultimately effects your beliefs that has an impact on your language, and so the cycle continues.

Language
- Positive
- Negative

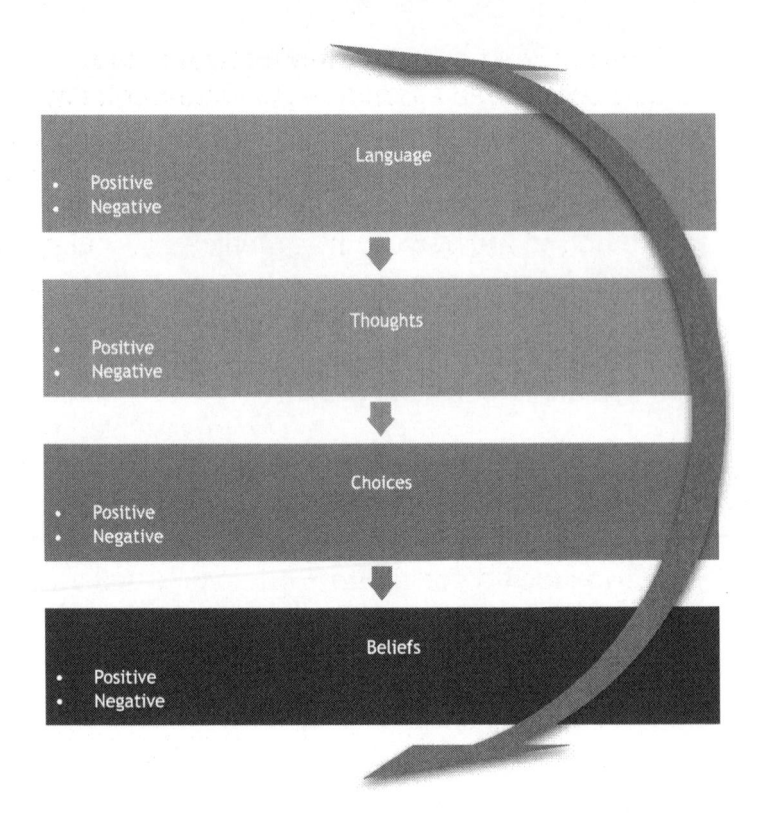

Thoughts
- Positive
- Negative

Choices
- Positive
- Negative

Beliefs
- Positive
- Negative

It is the same in most professional sports. I was working with a professional golfer on the European Tour, and he had a habit of going for the glory shot instead of playing the consistency game. Now there is nothing wrong with going for the glory shot IF you believe that you can make it. You see, this particular player didn't believe that he could make it and yet still went for it, which is suicidal in Golf.

We went for a round, and after 3 holes I said, 'don't hit the sand pit, it's just before the green.' You can probably guess what happened. Yep, straight in!

Once I explained what he was doing to himself, we worked on a strategy that has led to many successful tours.

Time and time again, I hear the self-sabotage in the language that people use around me, and although I'm tempted to correct them, I just smile to myself. You see, if you can recognise the negative language around you AND smile, then you are less likely to be affected by it. If you have spotted a mistake in someone's writing and you point it out to them, are they grateful and will they learn from it? The fact that you have found it means that YOU are less likely to make that mistake if that makes perfect sense.

I love those commercials and advertisements on billboards that are written to sell products, and yet they are written by professional people, being paid a huge sum of money to sell a product for their clients. I often wonder how much more they might have sold had they used a more positive language in their message.

When it comes to your habitual behaviours, listen to the language that you use and be careful what instructions you give your inner child. For example:

Write down some of the statements that you use about yourself and change them into more positive ones.

Negative statements	Positive statements	Negative statements	Positive statements
I'm starving	I could eat something		
I have always been fat	I am changing my size		
Could eat a scabby donkey	I could eat sensibly right now		
My backside is the size of a bus	I am changing my shape		
I can't stop eating	I choose to eat moderately		
I can't leave any food on my plate	I choose to leave a little		

For example: if you are always saying "I'm starving" then you are priming your brain to send messages of hunger to your body. If you were indeed starving then you wouldn't have eaten for 2-3 months.

Ask yourself "Am I really starving?"

When I hear people say that they want to 'lose weight', I begin to cringe for several reasons that I am going to share with you now. The effect that those two words have on the subconscious mind is disastrous as I'll explain.

The word 'loss' has a negative connotation on our beliefs because we are hardwired to avoid pain. Nothing positive ever comes from any statement that is preceded by the word 'lose'. People lose their jobs, loved ones, they lose money, self-respect, self-efficacy and confidence. Apart from weight, there is nothing positive about any statement that involves the word 'loss'.

Here are some neutral words that you can use instead of 'loss'. Let go, reduce, shed, stripped, dropped, taken off, ditched, etc. You get the message; these words will not have the same negative impact on your beliefs.

Whatever you focus on, you give energy to, albeit in cognitive form. Nonetheless, if you are considering quitting smoking and someone says to you how's the smoking going, what is the first thing that pops into your mind? Smoking!

It is the same with weight and whatever you give your energy to, it will somehow manifest itself into your world. Like debt, if all you are thinking about is getting out of debt, then you are focusing just on debt. So by thinking about weight in a generic form, you are indeed thinking yourself 'weightier'. Be really specific about the amount that you want to 'ditch' and when you make your goals, use that principle.

Delete the words 'lose' and 'weight' from your vocabulary and perhaps use something like: 'I will reduce my mass by 14lbs.' This way you are being really specific with your inner child and you are priming your brain with a positive statement.

Capture some of the negative statements that you make about yourself and then transpose them to a positive one.

Your potential

What is the definition of potential?

According to the English dictionary: Potential = Latent qualities or abilities that may be developed and lead to future success or usefulness - try changing some of your negative statements to positive.

The question I have is: How do you know what your qualities or abilities are?

Who determines HOW far you can go and what you can achieve?

Is it some mysterious force in the universe we call fate, or is it simply a matter of choices, determination and desire? You decide.

My personal opinion is that each of us has the ability to choose the language that we use unless you have Tourette's, a predisposition that affects the language filters that most of us use in a social situation, which means the person has no control over their language.

So unless you have Tourette's, you CAN choose the language that you use!

Put quite simply, YOU are the only one who gets to decide HOW far you can go, and it's a question of DESIRE, DETERMINATION and RESILIENCE.

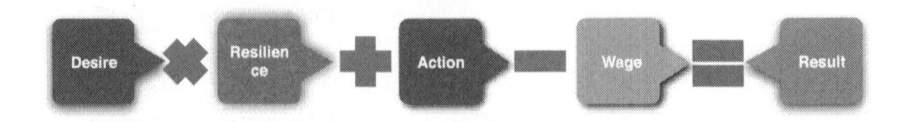

Desire ✕ Resilience + Action − Wage = Result

The only time that you get to fail is when you STOP and give up. When you get to that point, remember that you are almost certainly there, and achievement is just around the corner.

Remember this: 'Genius is 1% inspiration and 99% perspiration' ~ Thomas Edison, creator of the light bulb, amongst many other inventions.

There is an old proverb called '3 feet from gold'. It is said that during the gold rush era in the USA, one man spent everything that he had and found very little, until one day he eventually gave up! He sold his mine off to someone else for a very low price losing thousands of dollars. The man who bought the mine dug in it and, within three feet, found the biggest haul of gold ever recorded.

The moral of the story is to keep going even when you want to give up. If you have set your heart on becoming healthy and you give up 3 feet from gold, then you are programming your brain into believing that is acceptable to give up.

This means that you will never finish anything that you start because your story now becomes one of failure to complete. Regardless of how good your strategy is, if your story is weak, then you are less likely to get over the finish line and therefore stop 3 feet from gold.

The beauty of your brain is this: It only takes one success to smash that paradigm, and you begin to believe in yourself. It is the power in that belief in YOU that will get you over the finish line and find your gold.

If you were given a blank canvas and asked to DRAW the perfect picture of yourself, the person that you wanted to be, living the life you longed for, being surrounded by the people that you wanted and having everything you have ever desired, what would you DRAW? Your life is a blank canvas, and as from the day that you started to read this book, you have demonstrated a willingness to change something about you AND your life.

In Napoleon Hill's infamous book, 'Think and Grow Rich' (chapter 8), he dedicates a whole chapter to the importance of desire. In fact, he states that this is the single most important ingredient in the formula for success: When you want something so badly that, each morning you wake up, it is the first thing that you think about. When you are unable to get the thought out of your mind all day and you have an ache deep inside that just won't subside.

That is desire! If your desire is strong enough, you will find a way, and if it isn't, you will find an excuse. Feed your desire by allowing yourself to daydream about what it would be like to finally have what you have longed for. Imagine what people might say to you and who you would speak to first! How might you look and what would you be wearing in your mind's eye?

Resilience is a fascinating word and always makes me think of that famous quote by Sylvester Stallone in the movie Rocky: 'Let me tell you something you already know. The world ain't all sunshine and rainbows. It's a very mean and nasty place, and I don't care how tough you are, it will beat you to your knees and keep you there permanently if you let it. You, me, or nobody is gonna hit as hard as life. But it ain't about how hard ya hit. It's about how hard you can get hit and keep moving forward. How much you can take and keep moving forward. That's how winning is done!' I think this defines resilience perfectly.

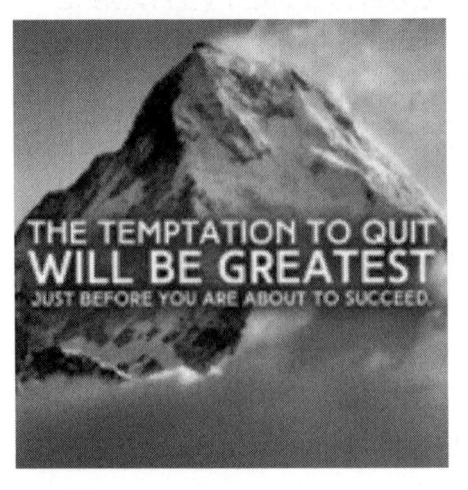

Applying action is the only way that we move something from our mind and make it real. Without action, your dream will only ever be a thought.

One of my favourite quotes is from Edward Everett Hale, an American author and Unitarian clergyman: 'I am only one, but I am one. I cannot do everything, but I can do something. And because I cannot do everything, I will not refuse to do the something that I can do.'

The moral is, as long as you are pointing in the right direction, each step or action, not matter how small, will take you closer to your desired outcome.

Keep moving forward, no matter how slowly, and at your own pace! The biggest mistake we make each day is to compare ourselves to others that are getting there quicker that we are. You will get there, no matter how long it takes you, and you will appreciate the journey and not just the destination.

The wage or price is paid in many forms – but the bill is always paid! – the toll it takes on you and those around you, the time that you have to invest, the money and self-development you have to endure and the endless hours of anxiety. Basic business understanding is that you have to remove your costs from your turnover before you can estimate your profits. The same in the equation above, only when you can extract the cost, can you say whether or not the result was indeed worth the investment.

The price is, of course, metaphoric in that, apart from the relatively small investment of exercise attire, it is monetarily free! It's the dedication required and the emotional investment that you make in sweat and hard work.

The results of winning or losing are, of course, a matter of choice and one that you alone can make. It is your path to follow, and nobody else can take that journey for you. If we made a movie of your life, would you be the main character in the story? If you are not playing the lead role in your life, then you are living in someone else's movie. Time to change the channel and become the very best version of you that shows up each and every day until they complete the journey that they have started here today. Choose to win because it will become a habit, and once that happens, you will reprogram your brain into believing that you ARE a winner.

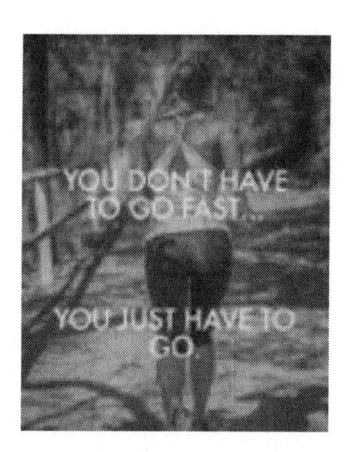

Summary

- Start your day from a place of gratitude and list all the things that you are grateful for in your life, no matter how small or insignificant you think they are. If you can't think of anything positive, then start with the fact that you are waking up because it is better than the alternative.

- Make a note of the stories that you are busy telling yourself and ask those around you to help you. Get them to point out each time you use one of those stories until you begin to recognise them yourself. It is time to change the channel in your mind, just like you would with a TV station that you are bored of. Make a list of the stories that you would like to tell yourself and read them each day.

- Does your strategy align with your desired goal or does it align with your story? Take a moment to look at your plan of action. Starting from the destination and working your way backwards to where you are right now in your life. Ask yourself, do I need to change my Strategy or my Story or both?

- Take special care with your language and leave out the negativity and influence it, instead, with positivity. Make a note of the negative things around you and leave some of them out of your life for 30 days, just to see if they make a difference. This may include some of your friends, especially if they are a fun sponge.

- Your potential is realised when your desire is multiplied by your resilience, plus the actions that you take: D.R.A.W.

- Remember to keep paying the toll in sweat by working hard, dedicate time to prepare your healthier meals and, most of all, be consistent.

Chapter 3
Thoughts

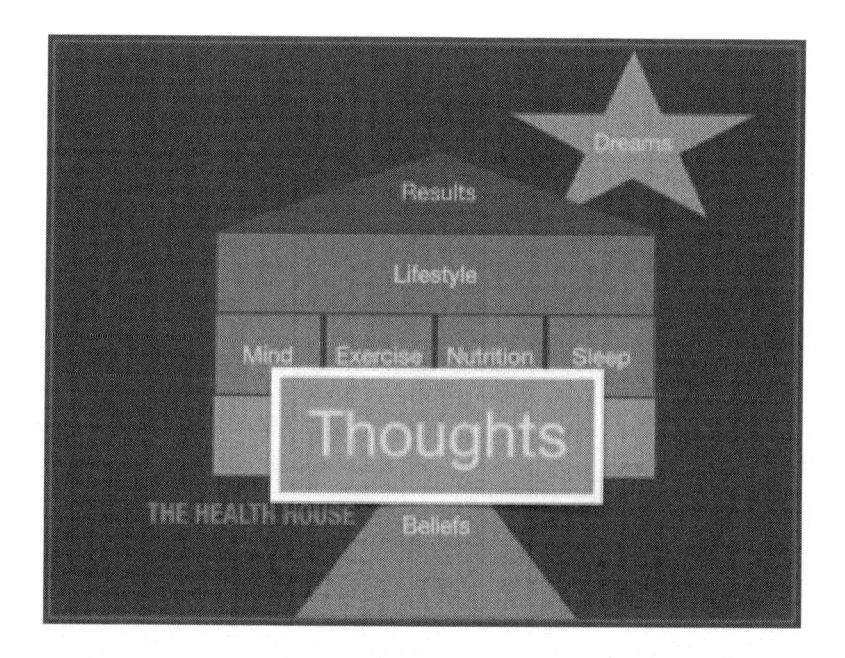

If our BELIEFS are underpinned by our VALUES, where do we get our values from?

There is scientific evidence that we get our values from a number of places, including:
- Parents - we can adopt the examples and opinions from our parents
- Environment - it includes your friends, school, social scene, etc.
- Genetic Pre-Disposition - the hardwired neural network of the brain

If you are one of the lucky ones AND you are happy with everything in your life including how you look, then you are one in a million that are already doing what I am about to suggest.

'Your subconscious mind is eavesdropping on your thoughts and acting accordingly.' ~ Deepak Chopra.

Deepak Chopra is an American author, and his books include 'quantum healing' and 'super brain'. He developed a way of harnessing the power of your thoughts to heal your own body of its afflictions from the inside out.

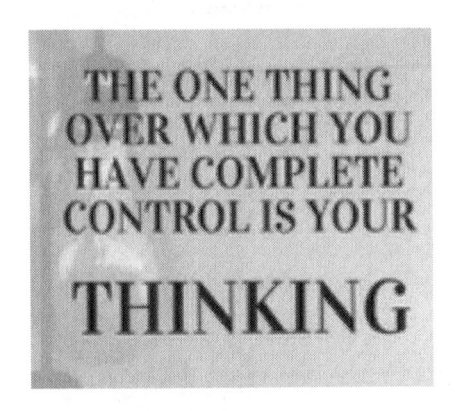

THE ONE THING OVER WHICH YOU HAVE COMPLETE CONTROL IS YOUR THINKING

The way that you THINK impacts upon what you believe, how you behave, how successful you are, how you feel, your confidence and ultimately your happiness.

Your THOUGHTS precede everything in your life, and you adjust yourself accordingly, mentally, physically and spiritually.

Change the way that you think and you change everything. Would you like to know the SECRET of how to make your thoughts work for you?
It starts with what you focus on AND the language that you use!

If you focus on all the things that you don't have, then you will never have them. If you come from a place of sincere GRATITUDE, then you are starting from a place that is both positive and powerful. Science argues that feeling grateful actually alters the neural networks in your brain AND affects how you FEEL.

By focusing on the things that you want in your life, rather than the things that you don't want, you are more likely to succeed in your ambitions, e.g. how many times have you heard someone say, 'I want to lose weight'? Probably a few, right? The very language suggests that the person is focusing on 'losing weight', which will have a negative impact on their thoughts and their success.

A more positive spin would be 'I want to become healthier.'

Let us review the thinking process in a human being. After all, once we can understand this, we can change it.

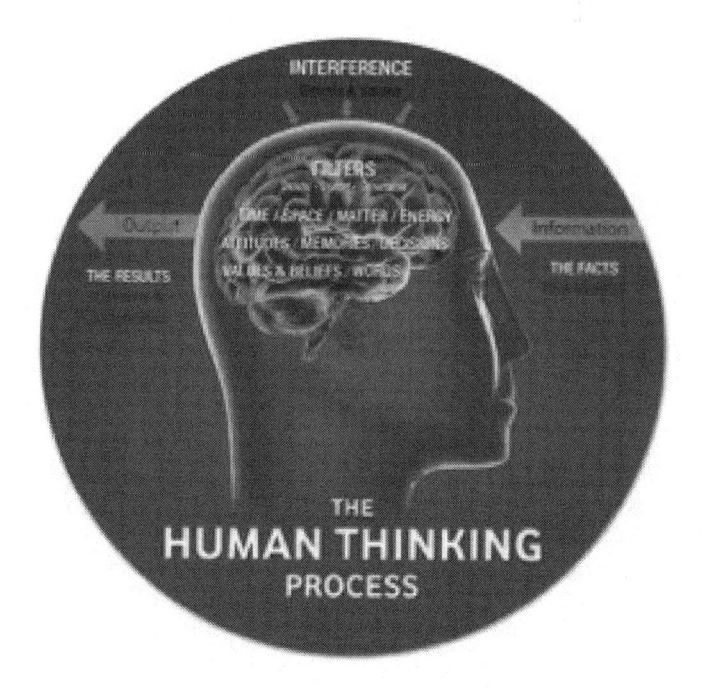

![The Human Thinking Process diagram showing a head in profile with INTERFERENCE at top, Information entering as THE FACTS on the right, FILTERS (TIME/SPACE/MATTER/ENERGY, ATTITUDES/MEMORIES/DECISIONS, VALUES & BELIEFS/WORDS) in the brain, and OUTPUT as THE RESULTS on the left]

As you can clearly see, information arrives from your sensory input, otherwise known as your senses: sight, sound, touch, smell and taste.

A little-known fact is that as you grow older, you choose a preferred way of receiving your information and then process it through filters before you make a decision.

Ask yourself what you see with. What do you hear with? What do you feel with? If you said anything other than you brain, then you, along with the majority of the population, would be wrong. It is your brain that allows you to see, hear and touch.

How does this affect what you do in life?

I am fairly confident that you have either said to yourself or heard someone else say, 'I want to get healthier but I just don't get the time to go to the gym.' Or 'I have worked so hard all week that I deserve to treat myself a little at the weekend.'

Years of experience in the sports and fitness world have taught me that a lot of these types of situations have taken many a strong willed gym buddy away from their goal.

I call this sort of thinking 'interference' because it interferes with your intention (thoughts) and your actions (behaviours) and it happens to even the very hardest minds in the business.

Matthew Yates in the '94 Olympics was tipped to be the greatest athlete with such high prospect, and the hope of the English nation rested on his young shoulders. He was consumed by the interference that he hadn't filtered out and dealt with that he didn't even make the starting blocks; instead, he couldn't make it out of the bathroom.

As a sport and exercise psychologist, I have come across this frequently, and the good news is there is a cure, and I'm going to share the secret with you right now.

Remember this:

Mental state + Choice +/- Interference = Results

Your current STATE of mind plus the CHOICES that you make, plus or minus the INTERFERENCE, equals the RESULTS that you get.

Ask yourself what is it that you are currently doing that is preventing you from achieving your goals? You need to show up every day to be the very best version of yourself to succeed in whatever you set your sights on.

Sometimes, you have to get yourself out of your own way to achieve greatness.

Your state of mind affects your entire being. Remember that your thoughts influence your language that in turn impacts how you feel.

> "A man is but the product of his thoughts. What he thinks, he becomes."
> *Mahatma Gandhi*

If you only take one thing from this whole book, then make it the following statement as this will definitely change your life if you apply it today:

You will become the accumulation of the thoughts and choices that you have made on a daily basis!

Your state is the term used for your current state of mind, your conscious thoughts and feelings that are happening right now.

Stop now and do a quick check:

Imagine for a moment that you have the biggest performance of your life, for the job that you have always dreamed of. How are you feeling right now?

Are your feelings positive? Where are they in your body, e.g. head, chest or stomach?

Now grab hold of your thoughts and stop them in order to evaluate what you were currently thinking for your body to generate those feelings.

Fact: Your body creates a somatic response to your thoughts! A significant emotional event (SEE) will trigger you to weigh up the current situation in your brain as it processes the information just like a computer would. When your brain has processed the information that it is presented with, then you make a subconscious choice to generate the feeling that you are now feeling.

If the event is significant enough and compartmentalised, it can have a detrimental effect on your beliefs that can result in low self-esteem, lack of self-confidence, unworthiness, overwhelm or anxiety.

Now that you know this, it should make controlling your thoughts really easy, right? Probably not, without practising a few thought control techniques first. Would you like to know more?

The good news is that there are plenty for you to practice as you read through this book. The diagram below shows how you choose to react to those feelings that are generated by your thoughts, which in turn cause interference and have a direct impact on your actions that has a direct effect on the results that you will get.

Maintaining a healthy state of mind is crucial to your daily success because it will ultimately impact upon the choices that you make, especially when it comes to what you eat.

Some Science For You

The choices that you make have an immediate effect on the way that you feel and, depending on HOW you choose to think, it will decide whether you allow interference to get in the way of your thinking.

Sometimes, you are your biggest critic, and for you to achieve your flow, you must get yourself out your own way.

Your brain creates pathways from the neurones (the building blocks of your brain and body's nervous system), dendrites (the branched extension of a neurone where electrical impulses are received) and synapses (the junction between two neurones where impulses are sent and received).

That is as much detail as we will need for the rest of the book.

What is really important to know is that it is much like a barcode on your favourite supermarket product. Your brain codes certain thoughts which in turn generate the feelings that you experience.

Now if you change one of the numbers on the barcode sequence, what happens? That's right, you get an entirely different product.

> "Patience, persistence and perspiration make an unbeatable combination for success."
> - Napoleon Hill

Well just like the barcode, if you change part of the sequence in your mind, you will get a completely different thought which in turn generates an entirely different feeling and therefore a different outcome.

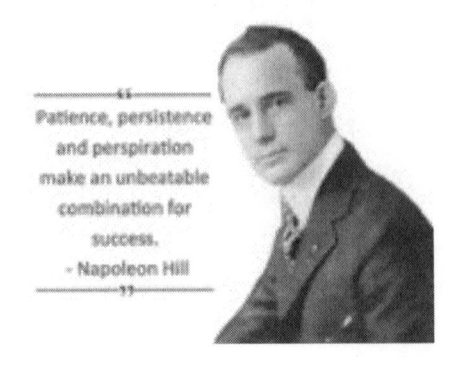

The neural pathways in your mind are just like walking through a forest, in the way that if you have a habitual response or strategy for dealing with a situation in a certain way, the more you think that way, the stronger the neural pathway becomes.

When you walk through a woodland or forest, and there is a path that others have walked previously, you tend to follow that pathway because it is easily marked out and easy to follow.

What happens when you start a new pathway in the woods and decide to walk through the foliage? The first few times are a little harder than the original path, but the more you walk the new course or create new neural pathways, the easier it will become as a process over time.

Getting into the brain is like getting into an exclusive nightclub where only the glamorous few are selected. Once inside, another gatekeeper, stress, determines what makes the cut to enter the upper VIP lounge in the prefrontal cortex

– that valuable 13% of cerebral architecture where our highest cognition and emotional reflection take place.

The brain evolved to promote the survival of the animal and the species. That means giving priority to a potential threat. Every second, of the millions of bits of sensory information from the eyes, ears, internal organs, skin, muscles, taste and smell receptors that are at the entry gate, only a few thousand make the cut.

The system that determines what gets in – what the brain attends to – is the Reticular Activating System or RAS. This primitive network of cells in the lower brainstem, through which all sensory input must pass to reach any higher regions of the brain, is essentially the same inside your dog, cat, child, and you.

The RAS favours intake of sights, sounds, smells and tactile sensations that are most critical to the survival of the animal and species. Priority goes to **CHANGES** in an animal or human's environment, especially the change that is appraised as threatening.

When a threat is perceived, the RAS automatically selects related sensory input and directs it to the lower brain where the instinctive response is not to think, but to react – **fight, flight, or freeze**.

When you are in a negative state of mind, HOW do you regain control of your thoughts and return to your positive state of mind? I mean things will happen on a daily basis that could affect your mood – if you let it.

For example, there will always be someone around that will cut you up in traffic or push in front of you in the queue, either your other half or your boss is in a foul mood, and it puts you on tenterhooks straight away, and so on.

Here is a little technique for you to practice, especially when you want to change a negative emotional state (mood) into a positive one:

Step 1

Your feelings generally move in particular directions. Direct your focus of attention to your belly and notice which direction your feeling is moving. It will be either:

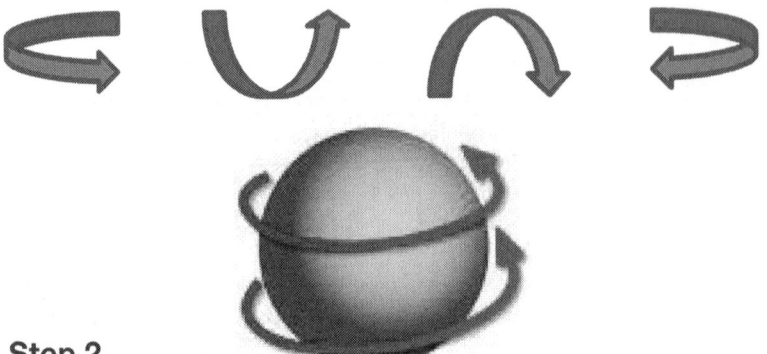

Step 2

Concentrate on that feeling and make it stronger. Rate it on a scale from 1 to 10 (1 being hardly anything and 10 being unbearable). Intensify it until it becomes a 10 on your scale.

Step 3

Using your power of imagination, take the feelings out of your body and, in your mind's eye, imagine it as a spinning ball of energy in front of you.

Step 4

Choose a **colour** that you most dislike and then imagine that the **ball** is now that **colour**.

Step 5

Now, this is critical. Stop the ball spinning altogether and then reverse the direction of the turn AND immediately change the **colour** to your **favourite colour**. Now that the ball is spinning in the opposite direction directly in front of you, notice what happens to the feeling, it should have dropped significantly down to a 3 or less. If not, repeat the process until this happens.

Step 6

Now you have a couple of options open to you:

- Do you want to keep the feeling?
- Do you want to get rid of it once and for all?

Step 7

Continue spinning the feeling and either snap it back into your body, in your mind's eye, or reduce the size of the ball to a marble size and imagine throwing it into orbit towards the sun where it will be obliterated once and for all.

You can find an audio version of this on our Facebook page or via our website www.leanbodyproject.co.uk available for you to download completely FREE. You can listen to the mp3 as many times as you want while you practice this amazing technique.

I still use this 'spinning' technique anytime that I find myself in a situation where I can sense negative and unwanted emotions beginning to manifest themselves.

A Bit More Science

In NLP (Neuro-Linguistic Programming), our reality and the world around us are run through a number of filters before we experience them in our minds.

These filters generate interference by deleting, distorting and generalising information that we receive from the outer world before it makes its way into our inner experience.

The deletion filter omits certain information, leading our minds to retain information only selectively. Not wanting to acknowledge parts of someone else's perspective is an example of this selective thinking process.

Likewise, you may not remember the exact shoes every person you spoke to today was wearing; your mind deleted the information from memory because it wasn't relevant.

If you intentionally wanted to remember every shoe colour and style of every person you met today, your mental filters might have worked differently, where you retained the information about shoes but perhaps deleted other details.

Our minds usually do not keep more than a specific amount of information at a time, making the deletion process somewhat necessary. The filter of distortion takes events from reality and distorts them based on our own perspectives.

For example, when a person sees healthy food, they can automatically say to themselves, 'it is going to be tasteless.' This is distortion just by looking at it. Only after taking a taste can the person actually make that decision.

Likewise, distortions can occur when we believe someone is trying to insult us when in reality they are not, and other situations where our perspective of the world attempts to overpower the actual objective experience of the world.

Generalisation works by taking a piece of information and generalising it to a category. The generalisation filter plays a role in aspects of our culture such as racism.

In therapy, the generalisation filter plays a role in looking at how we see 'the world versus me'. Often, when someone makes a remark, such as 'you are fat and ugly', we have a tendency to generalise this as the prevailing opinion of everyone in the world, rather than rationalising it down to a small and insignificant opinion of one person.

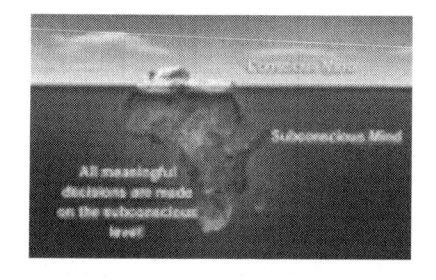

This is the reason that insults like this tend to hurt more than they ultimately do when we avoid generalising them. The purpose of the generalisation filter is to build the concept of 'reality' and 'world' in our minds; without it, we would have no such concept.

The beliefs and values that we have about the world influence the way that we use these filters in our lives.

Someone who is uncomfortable about receiving compliments from others may well delete every compliment he gets before it even makes it into his conscious mind. Likewise, a person who has a fear of flying on a plane may often distort their perspective on travel, heights, and even people who work for an airline because these factors are all based on their initial fear of flying.

Also, one who begins learning a new language and finds that the first thing someone in public says to them in that language is quite unpleasant may generalise the entire language to be fairly unpleasant.

Generalisations are not usually permanent, as we are constantly revisiting our concept of the world and what it means to be living in it.

I am always asked, 'how do you stop the interference from messing up your food choices?'

Well, there is more good news as preparation of food and planned daily exercise ritual is crucial to your success.

Remember that you CANNOT out train a bad diet!

Simplify your thought processes by planning a menu for the week, spend time preparing your food and schedule time for exercise – about 20 minutes a day will do.

By taking away the choice of what you FANCY eating and replacing it with 'THIS is what I am going to eat because I have already made it', will for most be the catalyst.

Next, make your thoughts work for you and set yourself up for success by writing some affirmations or statements of gratitude – 3-5 bullet points should do it.

An example would be 'Today I am grateful for waking up because it is better than the alternative' or 'I am feeling confident and looking forward to the day.'

Remember that you have already done the hard work before you even started your day.

By simplifying your thoughts and focusing on only three to five things daily, you will immediately influence your subconscious thoughts that impact on how you feel.

> Write your 3 statements here: i.e. Grateful or affirmations about you

You can join our Lean Body Project community by joining our Facebook group and share your statements to encourage and support yourself and others who are in the same boat as you.

If you allow the day to influence you in a negative way, and let's face it, we can all have bad days. It is how you respond to a particular incident that will define whether you are about to lose your temper or not.

Surround yourself with the things that make you smile, such as having a photo of your children or grandchildren in the car on the sun visor or on your desk at work. So that every time you begin to feel angry, you can look at the photo and reset your mood.

Have your favourite feelgood song in your cd player in the car or on your phone, so that you can listen to it when you need to lift your spirit.

You get the gist of this already, just have a backup plan that helps you.

Remember that your mental state, PLUS your choices, PLUS/MINUS interference equals the results (S + C +/- I = Results).

Summary:

- Remember that Generalisation, Deletion and Distortion are our brain filters that are based very much on our values, beliefs and, most importantly, our choices. When you make negative choices or doubt your ability, this is called interference.

- Your feelings of anxiety, doubt and worry are your body's way of telling your brain to change your thinking. Learn to listen to your body by noticing your feelings and then when you are in a similar situation, modify the barcode!

- Create your very own morning mantra that works for you and remember to say it out loud to yourself whilst looking in the mirror.

- Plan your meals in advance and pre-prepare them like a boss! It means that you have already planned what to do, which means that there is less chance of interference.

- It is important to know that you are in control of your thoughts and you have to process them first in order to have an emotional response (feel anything).

- Ask yourself what you can learn from the situation. There is always a learning point to any given situation, regardless of whether they worked out as you planned or not.

Chapter 4
Choices

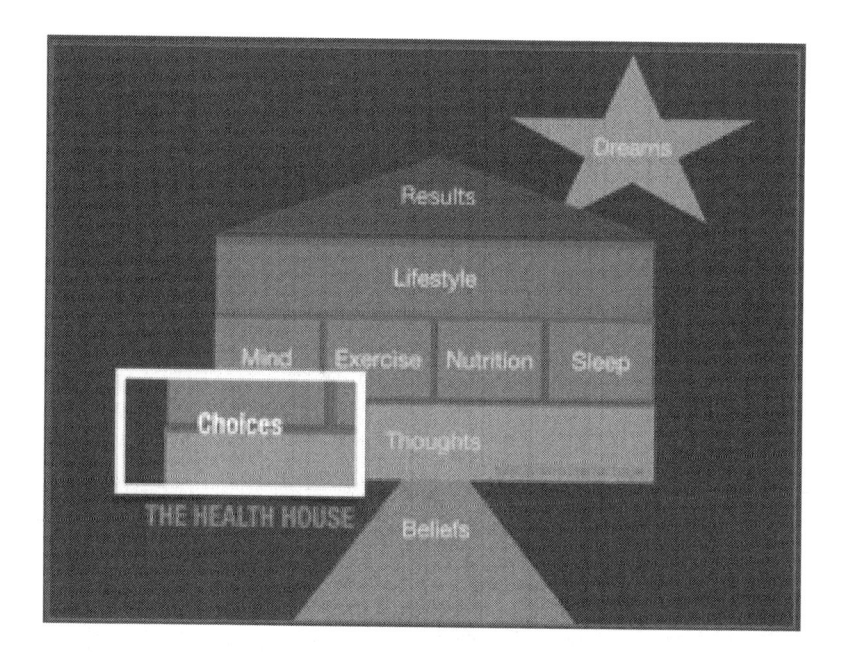

With respect to our health house, choices are the mortar that holds all the bricks together. You see if the building blocks are laid on the foundations of our beliefs and thoughts, then ALL the choices that we make will determine whether or not we achieve our goals.

You are where you are in your life right now due to the accumulation of choices that you have made on a daily basis.

Believe it or not, some people will categorically deny that they have had any involvement as to how their life has ended up. The first step to obtaining your goals is to take back control of your life! Most people get frustrated about their circumstances because they don't believe that they have any tangible choices left.

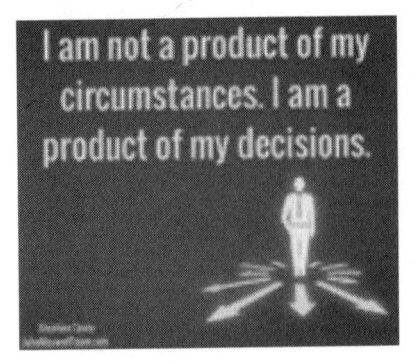

> I am not a product of my circumstances. I am a product of my decisions.

The reality of their situation, regardless of how dyer it may first appear, is that you always have a choice. The choice may be to do nothing, or make an investment, but there will always be a choice.

It reminds me of a story about two men laid up in the hospital both with terminal conditions. One of the men was near the window and the other one across the ward with only walls surrounding him.

As they began to get to know each other over a short period, the man near the window clearly had a more positive outlook on life as opposed to his friend that could only look at 3 walls.

The man near the window began to describe what he could see out of the window: 'A beautiful summer day overlooking a national park, the trees are bright and bursting with colour. Children playing whilst parents watch on. The grass is well manicured, and I can just make out a nearby football pitch. I can't wait until the weekend; we could watch them play.'
As both men were bed ridden, the man with only the walls to look at had to rely on his friend's commentary. As each day passed, the man with the walls for a view became increasingly jealous of his friend and he'd do anything to be able to have the bed near the window.

One night, the man near the window had a turn for the worst and begged his friend to call for the nurse. The other man stayed silent and pretended to be asleep. The next morning, he was woken by the commotion of nurses as they realised that the man next to the window had passed away during the night.

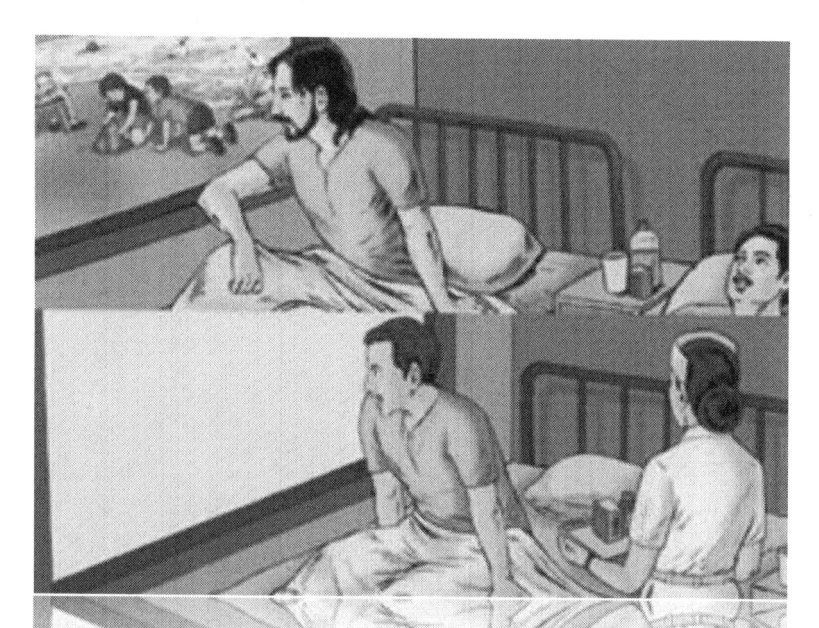

After the body had been moved and all evidence of his existence taken from the room, the man near the wall thought to himself that finally he'd get to be near the window and he asked the nurse if he could be moved to where his friend once was.

The nurse kindly obliged and moved his bed next to the window. Once the curtains had been opened, and to his horror, all he could see from the window was a brick wall of the adjoining ward, he died that very same night.

You see, the moral of this story is that it is not what you have in life, rather it is how you choose to see it. Just like the man in the story used his imagination to create a positive picture for his friend in the absence of any view.

Choice is such a powerful thing particularly when it comes to getting healthy and losing weight.

Some of our clients, when they first start with us, say, 'I have tried everything and I exercise every day. I just can't lose weight.' Which, might I state for the record, is an absolute crock of horlicks. If you have ever been ill with a tummy bug, such as this norovirus or gastric flu, then you will know that it is possible to lose weight (unless there is a specific medical condition).

On the 30 December 2016, the day before I was due to attend a New Years Eve party in Yorkshire UK, I started with a virus that laid me up in bed and as close to the amenities as was virtually possible. Over 5 days, I lost nearly a stone in weight. I wouldn't recommend this form of weight loss, nor would I wish it upon anybody because it is the most unpleasant.

The point I am making is that it IS possible to lose weight if you make the right choices and the necessary sacrifices for it.

'If nothing changes, then nothing changes.' ~ Jim Rohn

What people really mean is that they want to lose weight but they don't want to do anything different or change anything about their lifestyle, which means that their goal isn't going to happen.

In my experience, it is those choices that you make when you force yourself out of bed on a cold winter morning when it's raining or snowing outside, those days that you really don't want to go and put in the hard yards at the gym or the road work before you compete. Those will be the choices that will make the difference for you in the end and lead you to success or not.

I want to stress that the biggest myth in the fitness industry is that you can eat what you want providing that you burn it off in the gym. I often hear my friends say, 'I think that I'll have a pizza this evening because I'm playing football later and so I'll burn it off.'

NO! YOU CANNOT OUT TRAIN A BAD DIET!

Some of the biggest choices we can make are regarding what we put into our bodies in the form of nutrition. We either eat the wrong things or don't control portion sizes or feed cravings. Now to help you combat your cravings and give you a little more will power, it's first important to reflect on the underlying issue that is causing them.

One of the first exercises that I'd like you to do about this is to discover what type of overeater you are?

- Addictive eater
- Emotional eater
- Habitual eater
- Ignorant eater
- Destructive eater
- Angry eater

- **Addictive eaters** *crave sugary food, caffeine, junk food, colas and refined carbohydrates because they are addicted to the chemical composition of these foods. They always feel like these foods stimulate them to want more, and so they have great difficulty resisting them or eating just a little of this type of food.*

- **Emotional eaters** *find loneliness, boredom and sadness to be temporarily abated when they* *consume refined carbohydrates. After they fill their stomachs up quickly, they feel satisfied and sedated, even tranquilised, for a while. Comfort can briefly be found in soft sweet foods like ice-cream or cake that reminds us of childhood. Depressed people often want caffeine and sugary foods. Emotional eaters try to get rid of a bad feeling fast and feel good even faster by using comfort foods and bulk eating.*

- **Habitual eaters** *have often been made to eat everything on their plate. As children, they were often not allowed to leave food and have conditioned themselves to continue this habit. They will eat at every occasion and eat everything in front of them without being aware of whether they are hungry or not.*

- **Ignorant eaters** *have been completely brainwashed by food manufacturers to believe that what they are eating is healthy or harmless. They eat a lot of convenience and ready meals and believe they are as good as the home-cooked food. They may exist primarily on diet foods and diet drinks but still have a weight problem.*

- **Destructive eaters** *usually have a deep-rooted need to hide their sexuality and feel vulnerable when they look attractive or desirable. People who have never had enough, like volume and frequency of meals, that's why they always feel they may not get enough. They often feel panicky in a situation where food is shared, e.g. a group Chinese meal, in case they get less. They feel uncomfortable when they cannot dish out their own portions, but a host does it for them for fear of not getting enough to satisfy them.*

- **Angry eaters** *fancy crunchy food like crisps and apples and chewy food like meat and thick bread that they can chomp and chew on. Hard mastication is effective when we are feeling tense and wound up. Stressed people often want salty foods. They will always eat after a fight or disagreement to make themselves feel better.*

Identify which sort of eater you are, which one do you relate to the most. It is important to recognise the underlying driver that is making you eat so that we can provide you with a strategy for it.

If you would like to research this topic in more detail, then check out 'You can be thin, super-size vs super skinny' by Marisa Peer. In my opinion, there tends to be a deeper underlying issue that will require a more in depth strategy that is tailored to you individually.

One of the most powerful realisations and a good place to start if you are an "overeater" is to work out what triggers your compulsion to eat. Once you have identified your trigger food, then you can begin to create a strategy for coping with your urges when they arise. Note: If it is the environment, then you may have to either remove yourself from that environment or develop a good coping strategy.

Addictive eaters, I understand that this is not as easy as I am about to make it sound but rather than beating yourself up about your addictions, use them to your advantage and go with them rather than against them. Simply put, change the negative addictions to more positive ones, like going to the gym and eating healthier. After all, you weren't born having negative habits, you just learned them at some point and got used to them.

Emotional, angry and destructive eaters will need to deal with their emotions and own their thoughts, beliefs and language. Emotional eaters should feel nourished by things other than food. Angry eaters should express their feelings rather than eat them. Destructive eaters have an innate need to feel safe as well as looking good.

Ignorant and habitual eaters should aim to break their habitual emotional behaviours by recognising the patterns that trigger their compulsion and replacing them with healthy choices as we have explained in the previous chapter.

Remember that when you 'prohibit yourself' from having food, you will desire it even more. By changing HOW you communicate with yourself, you will change your cravings. Rather than saying to yourself, 'I am not allowed that pizza,' you can use 'I could have that pizza but I am choosing not to.'

You have a choice in everything in life and, although life has a way of provoking you when you least expect it, you will always OWN how you react or respond to those emotional experiences, which is a choice.

Scientists have discovered that the secret to actually following through with your well-intended decisions, is to remove EMOTION from the equation and therefore from your choices.

Remember, choices are like the mortar that binds the bricks of your house together. Your daily choices, however insignificant they may seem at the time will be the difference between success and failure.

I can remember the countless times that I have slowly dragged myself across to the edge of my bed at 5:30 am, still aching from the workout I had endured the day before. At that very moment in time, I have two choices:
A)   Jump out of bed and drag my weary be-hind to the gym

B) Turn over and have a snooze because missing one workout won't make too much of a difference

If I focus on the FEELING of aching and being tired, the likelyhood of me actually getting out of bed is significantly reduced by 50%. Here is a top tip of how to remove the emotion while doing a grocery shop.

Like most people in the UK, we tend to visit a BIG shop once a week, and we make a plan for all of our meals for that week. Why is this important and doesn't it seem a little OCD-ish?

Plan a (clean) healthy menu using the template below and then list all the ingredients that you will need to make those meals. Now add those ingredients to a shopping list, which means that you will be less likely to stray from your nutrition plan.

You'll find a template for you to use in the appendix of this book or online.

Monday
Tuesday
Wednesday
Thursday
Friday
Saturday
Sunday

Have you ever gone food shopping on your way home considering what you FEEL like eating for dinner? The chances are that you will FANCY something that will take you away from your goal, right?

Each day you will be faced with approximately 14,100 choices, and if you let your emotions interfere with your decision-making process, then you can probably guess what the outcome will be.

The crux of the matter is that you are where you are in your life due to the CHOICES THAT YOU HAVE made on a daily basis. If you don't like where you are right now, you need to make some different decisions.

Remember what Einstein said: 'the definition of madness is to keep doing the same things and expect a different result.'

If you applied one simple change to the choice that you make regarding your breakfast, for example, it may seem insignificant at first but over the period of 12 months, the difference will be incremental, and you will amaze yourself.

I'm what could be described as a fair weather golfer. I do however sometimes frequent the local driving range. When I stand on the tee and drive a ball over 200+ yards, I might hit 5/10 straight up the middle. Other times, I can send the ball over to the left or the right, depending on my grip and force.

When I hit the ball to the right, I know that I have pushed too much force through with my right arm rather than the natural swing of my hips. I also know that if I send the ball to the left that is because I have pulled too much force with my left arm or my grip was right.

Whatever the reason is, my club face only has to be out a tiny fraction for the ball to go astray. A small misalignment in the club face won't do much to the trajectory of the ball over 10-20 yards, but over 200 yards, it could be a long way off target.

When we make some small insignificant choices of indulging, such as having a sneaky packet of crisps or a bar of chocolate, cake or packet of sweets, no one will ever know, and in the short term, it won't make a huge difference, but over the period of a month or even a year, it will have a massive effect on both our weight and our health.

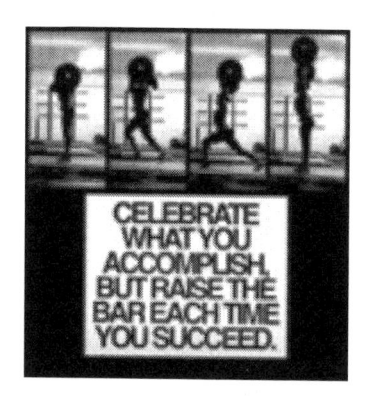

CELEBRATE WHAT YOU ACCOMPLISH, BUT RAISE THE BAR EACH TIME YOU SUCCEED.

That one extra beer or glass of wine that you won't miss if you were to just cut it out, what difference would that make to you in years' time?

Small choices add up and become significant changes and big results.
Choices and indecision are only difficult until they become ingrained into our subconscious, and then they become habits.

Once those new selections have become habitual daily behaviours, then it becomes easier to cope with some of those potential situations that trigger a compulsion. The key is to develop between 2-5 new behaviours per week so that it is not too much of a shock for your system and avoid overwhelm.

Write down what your biggest challenges are when it comes to getting healthy and be specific as to what your main barriers are.

My biggest challenges are:

Being really honest with yourself, what advice would you give to a friend if they were in your situation and you were listening to them?

Plan out all the behaviours that you are going to adopt over the next 28 days and list which ones you will change in which week.

One of the biggest main challenges for most of our clients is the WEEKEND. For whatever reason, most people go into the weekend on auto pilot where normal service is resumed. That, of course, comes with a cost attached to it, in the form of 72 hours.

When your body consumes alcohol for example, which is very high in sugar, it takes up to 72 hours for it to get out of your system. This means that your body will burn the sugar and the effects of the alcohol first before it begins to burn fat.

So, someone enjoying the weekend Friday, Saturday and Sunday, it will be at least Thursday before their body begins to burn fat again, and then it's Friday the next day, and so an endless harmful cycle begins.

The choice that you have to make is this: Are you where you want to be with your health and body shape? If yes, then go ahead and maintain your silhouette. If no, then you need to make different decisions, particularly going into the weekend.

For me, it's simple: you are either ON plan or NOT and if you are cheating at the weekend, then the only person that you are cheating is you. Be honest with yourself starting from now.

If you are going to a party, wedding, birthday or night out with friends, providing you can accept the fact that you are cutting yourself some slack but getting straight back on it the next day, then go for it. Life is for living after all and, providing that you are on it 80% of the time, you should do ok.

My main concern is that you don't feel guilty about having an one-off indulgence, providing that it is not every weekend. If you have major guilty feelings afterwards, then you may need some additional coaching.

One of my favourite times to let your hair down is on holiday. Some might not agree with me when I say that it's okay to completely let your hair down on holiday.

The reason for this is that it is exactly what it is: a holiday from the daily routines that allows you to completely relax for 10-14 days. If you've worked hard all year, then you have earned it in my book.

Rest is as good as a change, and recharging your batteries both emotionally, physically and mentally is absolutely crucial in your journey, and it is always a good motivator to attain your beach body.

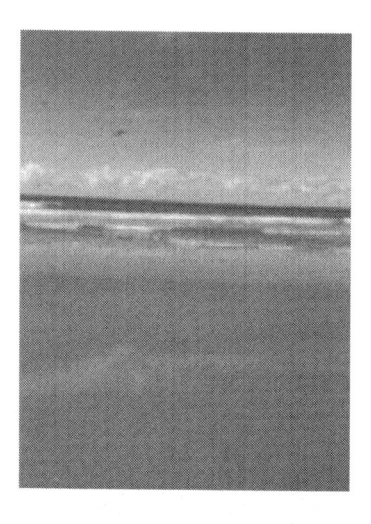

Mind

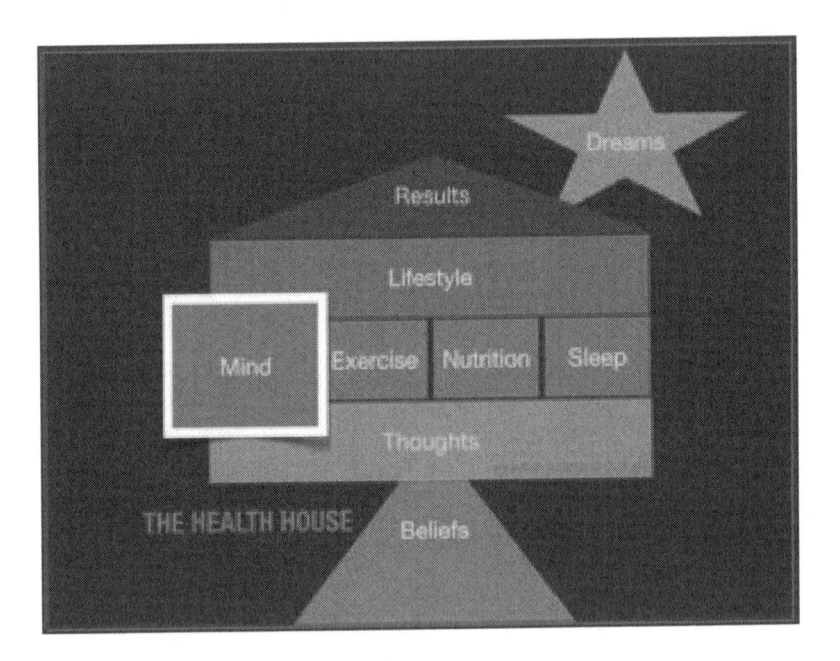

[The Health House diagram: Dreams (star), Results, Lifestyle, Mind (highlighted), Exercise, Nutrition, Sleep, Thoughts, Beliefs]

Your mindset is the first one of our bricks in the health house, and it serves to remind us that unless we get this particular bit right first, it will be like building a house using bricks that crumble.

I previously mentioned how your thoughts can impact upon your subconscious mind and, providing you are really specific with your language and purposeful with your thoughts, you can develop the right mindset.

If you compare your subconscious mind to a 4-year-old and then treat it as such, you will find that it can start to work for you rather than against you. If you were to call a friend on the land line and their 4-year-old picked up the phone, what would you say?

If you asked them, 'Is your mummy home?' what would the response most likely to be? A standard 'yes', and the likelihood of them taking the phone to mummy would be very remote. That is unless you are really specific and say, 'Is your mummy home and can you take the phone to mummy?' The chances of them passing the phone to mummy have just increased by about 80%.

Your subconscious mind works in the very same way and, let me tell you that from experience, it is the first thing that you need to get right. You see, you can have the best exercise and nutritional program in the world but without preparing your mind first, it will most likely fail.

It has been my privilege to work with some of the very best athletes at the very top of their games over the years. I can remember a friend that was training for an Iron Man event.

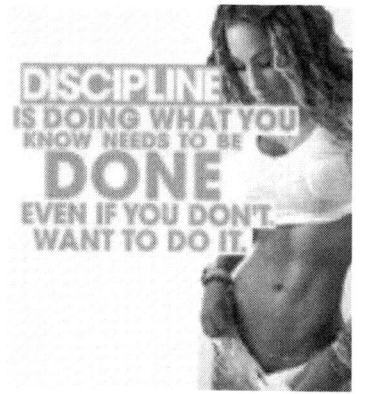

This is an event that is set over a 2.5-mile swim in open water, followed by an 112-mile cycle ride and finishes with a full marathon of 26 miles.

We worked together to develop an athlete's mindset which involves daily discipline that is created through pure persistence and sometimes forcing yourself to do the things that you really do not want to.

For example, getting up at 5 am to cycle 12 miles on a cold winter morning. At 5 am at minus 5 and during a blizzard, I can understand that your inner child would be screaming at the top of its voice. It would have been having a tantrum and shouting, 'I don't want to get up out of bed, its cold and it's the middle of the night.' It takes a lot of willpower and discipline to ignore the inner child and just get on with it.

Sometimes, it's those dark days when you are laying in your bed and the alarm goes off and the last thing that you want to do is get up. You may need some extra support, which is where the people that you have around become crucial. I would get up at 5 am and call my friend because I knew that if I didn't, he wouldn't have trained. I would stay on the phone with him all the way around his 12 miles which could be up to 40 minutes or so.

It took dedication and commitment on both our parts, and I'm delighted to say that, after 12 months of training, he completed the course and in just over 15 hours. To qualify for Iron Man, you have to finish the course in under 16 hours too.

Here's how you can transform your mindset from an inner child to an athlete:

1. List 21 things that you have done successfully throughout your life
2. Place them on a timeline of your life (see diagram on the next page)
3. Delete the T from Can't
4. Shut the 'duck' up
5. Put the child on the step
6. Visual motivation

As we have stated in the previous chapters, your subconscious mind is directly influenced by your conscious mind. The conscious mind is currently taking in the present

```
┌─────────────────────────────────────────┐
│  21 things that I have achieved in my life: │
│                                         │
│                                         │
│                                         │
│                                         │
└─────────────────────────────────────────┘
```

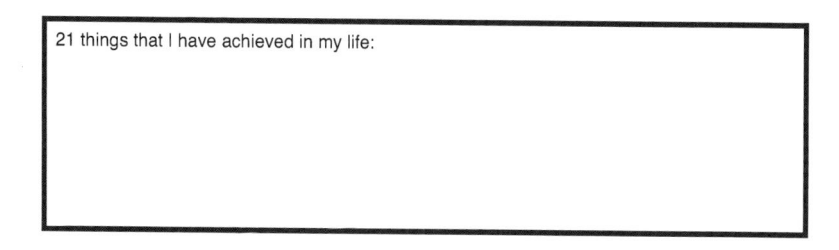

situation – it includes your self-talk and any interactions. Your subconscious mind is reportedly somewhere below your neck region and should not be confused with the unconscious mind which is pretty much when someone is in a coma.

Your conscious mind which includes your decision making is also directly influenced by your innermost thoughts. For example, when the alarm clock goes off, and you say to yourself, 'I can't be bothered going to the gym,' and 'It's only one workout, it won't make much of a difference.'

This is your inner child or innermost thoughts influencing your commitment to your fitness regime. It might not make too much difference if you are feeling unwell or it's a recovery day. The trouble is, that since your inner child has won once, it will try again and again. This means that you will probably repeat this behaviour and if that becomes a habit, then it WILL make a difference!

Now make a list of the things that you have achieved in your life up until now, regardless of how insignificant you think that they are:

Make your timeline from 0 to 100, which signifies the day you were born to 100 years old. Now mark off half way (50)

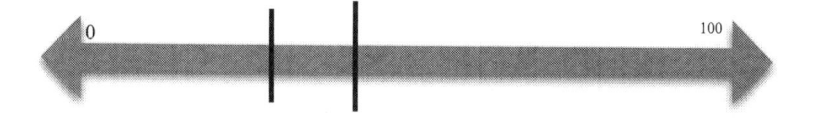

⟵―――|―|―――――――――⟶
 0   100

and now add your age, mine's 45 and begin to populate it with your achievements.

It doesn't have to be exact; an approximation will do. Now begin to write in your achievements at the age that you were when you accomplished them.

So the example above shows that I am currently 45 years old and I contracted viral meningitis when I was 30 years old. This proved to be a catalyst in my life because it made me reassess everything and prioritise the things that were most important to me.

I no longer saved my best wines for a special occasion, in fact, I would invite people around to the house just so I could open one. It is amazing how near death experiences can change your perspective on life.

My bucket list wasn't going to be put off until I had retired and I could effectively afford it. I was going to make things happen and forge ahead with fulfilling my dreams. It is the most liberating feeling in the world when you can adjust your mindset and free yourself from the shackles of self-limiting beliefs.

Realising that you have achieved so much already in your life in such a short period should be a reminder that you can make anything happen when you really apply yourself. Remember back to one of those achievements in your mind's eye and ask yourself what the difference maker was for you. What were you doing differently back then that you could be doing now?

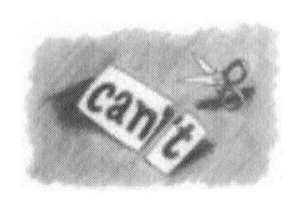

We have already mentioned earlier in the book about deleting the 'T' and highlighted the only difference between can and can't is the T, so lets get rid of it.

Whenever you hear either yourself or someone else say the words 'I Can't', you need to help them reframe the situation and respond by helping them delete the 'T.'

Jessica Ennis-Hill, one of the UK's most successful and decorated track and field athletes, first won the gold in the heptathlon 2009, again in 2010, 2012 and 2015, and before retiring in 2016, she managed to achieve silver in the Rio Olympics.

It has been widely reported, but particularly by Dr Steven Peters, that when Jessica is warming up on the track before her events, she has a tendency to let doubt creep into her mind and say things to herself like 'what are you doing here? With all these brilliant athletes, who do think that you are?'

Jessica has a 'coping strategy' by which she will imagine that the negative self-talk is coming from a duck that is sat on her shoulder. Her response to that duck is, 'shut the duck up.'

When you are next in a position where you are doubting yourself, even if it is during an exercise class or getting out of bed in the morning, what mantra can you conceive that will help you turn down the volume on that inner voice and put the child back in its place?

When the self doubts come in to play, I want you to have a plethora of affirmations about yourself at the ready, so that we can put the inner child on a naughty step. It will be a constant battle between you and that child until you develop your strategy into a daily habit. This requires effort at first, but you will soon get into the swing of things.

Write a list of affirmations about yourself, say about 10 or so and remember to include some things that you are grateful for too. Repeat these each morning as you awake. You don't have to shout them out loud or say them in the mirror as long as you say them in your head every day.

As soon as you recognise the inner child spitting out its dummy (or pacifier), that's your cue to start your mantra until you can no longer hear the negativity.

Finally, in your success strategy there is an adaptation of the 'cheque' from 'The Secret' by Rhonda Byrne, where you write yourself a cheque for the amount that you want and you stick it to the ceiling above your bed. So it is the first thing that you see when you awaken and the last thing that you see before you sleep.

First, ask yourself if you are motivated by pleasure or pain. This is not a sadistic exercise, it is merely to identify if you are driven towards pleasure and gratification or away from pain. Only YOU know and be honest with yourself.

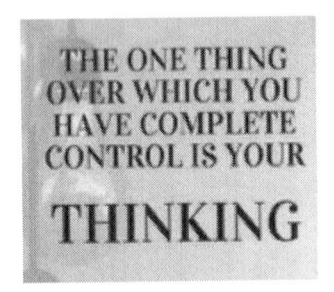

> THE ONE THING OVER WHICH YOU HAVE COMPLETE CONTROL IS YOUR THINKING

If you are motivated towards achieving your goals, then place a photo of HOW you would like to look. This can be an old photo or one that you have photoshopped or, alternatively, one cut out of a magazine.

If you are motivated away from pain, then place a picture of you in your worst shape. You know that one photo that was the catalyst and made you take action because you can't stand how you looked.

Place them above the bed on the ceiling or on the bedside cabinet, or put them on the refrigerator door to remind you of your goal each time you reach for something to eat and spur you to make the right choices for you.

In conclusion, creating your athlete mindset:

Time: up to 28 days, if you are serious.
Desire: at all times, remind yourself why you are doing it with the visual motivators.
Resilience: repeating your affirmations each morning will help you develop this.
Actions: you will need to ditch the interference of the inner child and apply action.
Wage: the price is daily discipline until you get where you want to be.

Start by taking control of your own happiness.

You have got to be IN it to win it! You can't expect to do this half-heartedly and expect great results. Develop yourself and invest in your mind. Set your mindset for the day as soon as you wake up and don't leave it to chance or for someone else to brighten your day.

How many people do you know that are all too willing to take care of their bodies and their finances BUT willing to leave their MINDS unprotected?

Let me explain. If we spent as much time pre-preparing what we feed our mind and exercising the biggest muscle that we have (our brain), then everything else would fall in line.

Examine your morning routine for a second and look at what you do from the moment that you open your eyes to when you leave the house.

Now list everything that you have to think about! There won't be many, right?

If you meander through your morning routine, influenced by anything and everything around you, then you are setting yourself up for FAILURE.

What if there was a way to KICK START your day that actually sets you up for SUCCESS?

Well, there is:
- When your alarm goes off, get up straight away and ditch the snooze.
- Start your morning from a place of gratitude.
- Drink a glass of water after you have brushed your teeth.
- Set some time apart for reading – just 10 pages a day will suffice.
- Work out what you want to achieve for the day in order for you to feel productive.
- Exercise – just 20 minutes of exercise per day will have a significant impact on how you think.

Look after your mind because your body is a slave to it, be careful what you feed it. Eat foods that are also good for your brain because the first battle you have to win when it comes to getting healthy is in YOUR mind.

There is substantial evidence that suggests that we are the accumulation of the 5 people whom we spend the most time with. Think of the traits and habits of some of your closest friends and family and ask yourself if they are ADDING to or taking you AWAY from your goals.

If you are serious about becoming healthy, then you might have to examine who you spend the most time with.

Make your morning routine work for you and don't leave it to chance AND be prepared to cull those around you until you reach your goals.

A great book to read on the subject is 'Miracle Morning' by Hal Elrod.

If you have read the book and tried the miracle morning for yourself, share your thoughts on the subject, and have the freedom to post in the Lean Body Project Facebook group.

Check out the appendix for our daily planner templates.

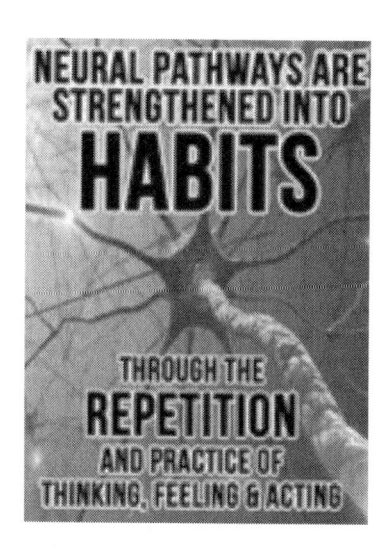

NEURAL PATHWAYS ARE STRENGTHENED INTO HABITS THROUGH THE REPETITION AND PRACTICE OF THINKING, FEELING & ACTING

Exercise

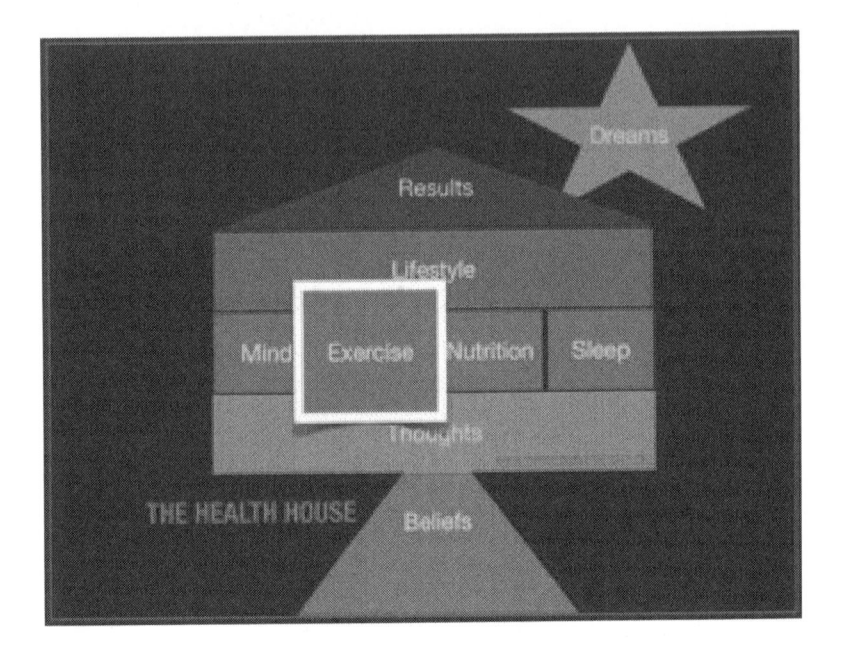

[Diagram: The Health House — showing building blocks labeled Mind, Exercise (highlighted), Nutrition, Sleep, with Lifestyle above, Thoughts and Beliefs as foundation, Results as the roof, and Dreams as a star above.]

The physical benefits of exercise are well documented and have been for centuries. We tend to accept that engaging in regular exercise is something that we SHOULD do but often choose not to.

If this is the case, WHY is it that we are unable to motivate ourselves to get active on a regular basis?

The mental benefits of regular exercise go far beyond the realms of just getting rid of the dreaded beer belly or the muffin tops. In fact, there is strong evidence to suggest that participating in as little as 20 minutes high-intensity training on a regular basis can significantly reduce the risk of mental illness.

If doctors were to prescribe regular exercise as opposed to drugs in the treatment of depression or anxiety, we would save the NHS a small fortune.

The body has its own method of balancing the hormones, which is all controlled by the 'Master Gland' (Pituitary) which is located at the base of our brain.

When our body is lacking a hormone, the brain tells the body to produce more and when it has too much, it also orders it to stop.

Have you ever wondered why we feel so good after exercise? This is because our brain tells our body to produce the FEEL-GOOD hormones called endorphins during exercise. These hormones are used by the body to dull pain, combat depression and anxiety, reduce stress, and improve sleep and self-esteem.

Now for the curve ball! How do you currently exercise your brain?

According to an article on Neurogenesis in the New Scientist published in the Guardian newspaper, an active mind, when properly stimulated is capable of producing new brain cells even in people that are 125+ years old.

Anything that stimulates your mind enough to THINK about something such as reading, problem-solving, puzzles, board games and conversation are all proven ways to keep your mind sharp.

There are many versions of 'brain gym' that will promote cognitive 'whole brain thinking' by engaging both its hemispheres and lift the limits of the 'neural highway' otherwise known as the 'corpus callosum'.

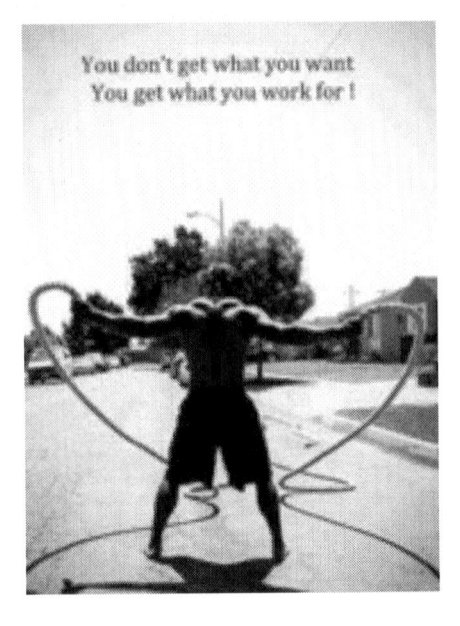

If 20 minutes of physical exercise is now accepted to prolong our life span, then 20 minutes MUST be recommended to maintain our mental faculties.

Just 20 minutes is also said to help us get a better night's sleep. According to a recent study by Appalachian State University, morning workouts are ideal if you want the best night's sleep. The study found that those who exercised in the morning (7 am) slept longer and deeper than their counterparts that exercised during the day.

This is the part that almost everybody gets wrong.

Whenever they start out with a new fitness and 'weight loss' goal, more often than not they will join a gym or fitness class and punish themselves for a while with little to no results and then fall off the waggon.

As I already mentioned, exercise is awesome, but on its own, it has been shown to be pretty ineffective for weight loss and actually increases hunger, this is why the exercise more and eat less thing is a bad idea.

However, the right kind of exercise along with the right kind of nutrition plan can help you achieve amazing results – praise the Lord!

Now you may notice that I said 'the right exercise', so let me explain a little.

Of course, any exercise is better than no exercise, but I'm guessing you want to know how to achieve the best results in the fastest time, right? Yes, I thought so.

Most people when they decide to start working out to lose weight, they think that they need to do lots of cardio, right? Sorry to tell you, but you're wrong.

Cardio exercise is great for your heart and lungs and also for your fitness, but it's not the best thing you can do to help you get in shape, lose body fat and get toned unless you are severely obese and out of shape. Then yes, it would probably be best if you started with some degree of low-intensity cardio and just generally moved more.

Nine times out of ten, people want to lose weight and get toned, yet they spend all of their time doing cardio and not doing any toning. Sounds silly when you hear that, doesn't it?

Doing this will only end up with you looking 'skinny fat' – which is just a smaller version of what you were before.

To get in shape and tone up, it's important that you maintain muscle, not burn it away.

Muscle is more metabolically active than fat, meaning that the more lean muscle you have, the more calories you will burn while you sit on your backside.

Therefore, it makes much more sense to help preserve what little muscle you might have and even focus your training on using that muscle so that you can burn more fat and sit on your backside more.

I call this thinking smarter not harder and if there is a shortcut to getting in shape, then you, as well as I, want to be clued up on it so we can use it to our advantage.

I just want to make something very clear: cardio isn't the best thing you can do for fat loss – maybe you have already figured this out with your own frustration.

High-Intensity Interval Training (HIIT), on the other hand, is much better and gives you all the benefits and more than typical traditional cardio.

Some fans of cardio get upset with me when I tell them this, but I'm not saying, 'Don't ever do cardio,' I'm just telling you what's best to get results.

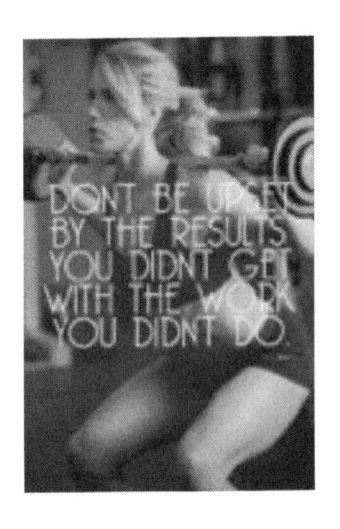

If you like to go for the occasional run as I do, then go for it, just don't use traditional cardio as your main tool to getting lean.

Traditional cardio can increase cortisol levels, which can actually prevent you from losing weight and possibly even gain weight, and we don't want that.

I like to go for an occasional run to clear my head and to help de-stress sometimes, or if the weather is nice, I tend to get outside for a few runs.

If you happen to like running, keep it up but try adding in some of the HIIT workouts and weight training as well, and you will probably see an improvement in your fat loss results.

HIIT Training

Now, what's so great about HIIT training then?

Well, depending on what exercises you do, it's like killing two birds with one stone, e.g. if you are doing a body weight circuit including press ups, squats, burpees and planks, then you are adding resistance to your muscles which will help to tone and firm them while burning fat.

Also, you will notice that it's very challenging fitness-wise even more so than traditional cardio.

How? Because with regular cardio, you generally only go at one stable and steady pace. With HIIT, you are keeping things fast-paced and using many different exercises and methods all at a high intensity.

Workouts, therefore, don't need to be as long, and the overall fat burn effect is much better.

This is something called the After Burn Effect or the proper terms for this is EPOC which stands for 'Excess Post

Oxygen Consumption'. It has been shown to keep burning body fat for up to 48 hours.

Cool, right? So, when it comes to cardio training, think smarter not harder.

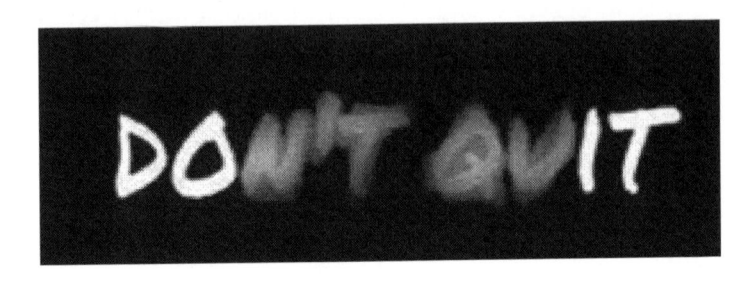

Bodyweight Training

Body weight training is awesome because you don't even need a gym. You can train in the comfort of your own home or outside in the park, literally anywhere. You don't need expensive equipment.

And you don't need to train for hours at a time unless you are training for a sport or an event.

Some of my online programs are based around doing only 10-minute bodyweight HIIT circuits at home, and the results are amazing.

Don't underestimate the effect of a daily 10-minute workout. I have hundreds, if not thousands, of before-and-after pictures and screenshots of some amazing results.

Sometimes for a very well trained person, a sportsperson or athlete for example, obviously 10 minutes are probably not going to be enough.

But consistency is the key. It's better to do 10 minutes a day, every day, than only one 60-minute workout per week.

Of course, the fitter you get, the more time and intensity you can add onto the workouts, and I would definitely encourage this, but don't use time as an excuse not to be able to workout when you can smash out a quick 10-minute home workout.

Bodyweight training is great but this may only take you so far, long term and as with anything, you should always be looking to progress.

The natural progression from bodyweight would be weight training.

Weight Training

Weight training is often avoided by women for fear of that it's going to make them look like a Russian shot putter. Trust me, this is never in a million years going to happen.

Mostly all of the bodybuilding pictures you see will be using some kind of steroids or synthetic enhancement.

Not only this, but they will have most likely dedicated years and years of training and strict nutrition with very little social life.

This is their 'game'. This is what they train for over time to be competitive in that sport. To compete in any sport, you have to be prepared to make sacrifices, but the level these athletes go to is next level, way beyond what the average person wants or needs to do to achieve a nice toned, healthy looking physique.

There are many guys out there, myself included, that train seriously hard and eat well but still don't get massive, so there really is no reason to be scared of lifting weights.

Women produce about 50% less testosterone than guys do, so it's almost impossible to get huge and bulky without some sort of synthetic assistance, a life dedicated to lifting weights and a shrine in your bedroom worshipping Arnold Schwarzenegger.

Instead, you will look lean and toned, firm and sexy and you will feel more confident and ultimately be happier.

Sprint Training

Sprint training is awesome!

Have you ever seen the body and shape of a sprinter?

Male or female, their bodies are lean and toned.

It's all down to the way they train, and of course how they eat – but remember they are professionals, so they eat, sleep and train a hell of a lot more than what we 'ordinary people' do.

If you want to look like an athlete, then you need to do what athletes do.

Athletes have to make many sacrifices while they are training, including social events, but they still have to eat clean and train hard all the time whether they are having a good day or not. If their mood dips or they just can't be bothered, then it's tough because they still have to do it. They still have to work on themselves to achieve the result they want. No excuses.

We could all learn a thing or two from the mindset of an athlete.

Sprint training is a form of cardio training but far superior to traditional cardio on the most part.

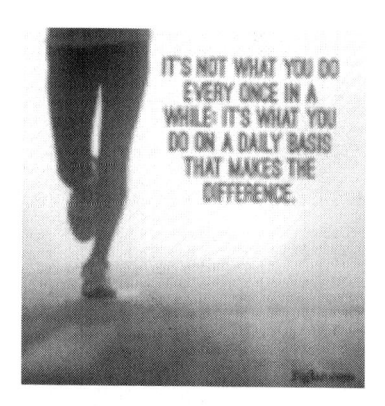

Sprint training uses the anaerobic energy system, whereas traditional cardio uses the aerobic system.

Anaerobic means 'without oxygen', hence we can only sprint over short distances before we need to rest and recover.

The more we can train in the anaerobic system, the more energy we burn and overall more body fat.

You should make sure that you are properly warmed up beforehand and build yourself up with a few shorter and less intense sprints first. You don't want to be diving straight into maximal sprints without having a good warmup unless you want to give yourself an injury.

Sprinting is very taxing on the body so when you are just starting out, you should probably only start with a few and then gradually build up.

Simply set yourself a distance like 50-100 meters and then sprint from start to finish, walk back slowly till you are fully recovered and then repeat 3-5 times and gradually build on this over time. If you are running on a treadmill or using another piece of cardio kit in the gym, you could do 30 to 60-second sprints, taking the equivalent time to recover with a more moderate pace.

Nutrition

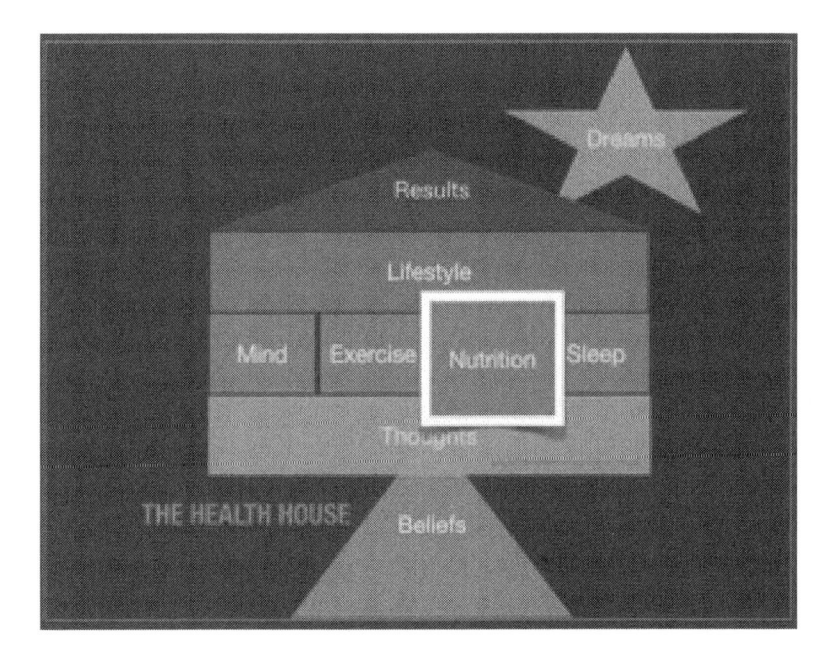

[Diagram: The Health House — a house shape with Dreams (star), Results (roof), Lifestyle, with Mind, Exercise, Nutrition (highlighted), Sleep, Thoughts, and Beliefs as the foundation.]

Ever heard the expression 'you are what you eat'? Well, it is certainly true when it comes to the wellbeing of your MIND as well as your BODY.

According to the National Centre for Health Statistics and the Office of National Statistics UK, people are living longer than the previous generation and subsequently expand their lifespan in line with modern medicine.

The messages regarding nutrition that we receive through the power of the media are so mixed and tend to be subject to change within such a short space of time.

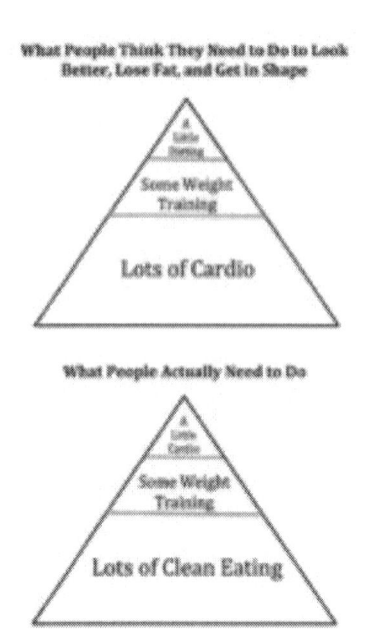

What People Think They Need to Do to Look Better, Lose Fat, and Get in Shape

- A Little Dieting
- Some Weight Training
- Lots of Cardio

What People Actually Need to Do

- A Little Cardio
- Some Weight Training
- Lots of Clean Eating

As a red wine drinker, I was delighted to learn that a small glass with food is PROVEN to be beneficial to one's health. The very next day it was deemed to be the exact opposite and recommended limits should be 7-14 units of alcohol per week.

There was such a famous debate during the 1980's when EGGS were given a rough ride due to the risk of salmonella, and now the world's medical profession promote them as the next super food and every day should begin with a staple diet of eggs.

What we might be aware of is the fact that our bodies crave nutrients and NOT FOOD! This is driven by the body's survival mechanism to ask for whatever mineral or vitamin it is lacking.

The body sends a message to the brain where it is processed through a series of internal filters until a decision of desire is reached.

If we are living longer and looking after our bodies better so that we can still remain independent in our old age, what are we doing to ensure that we remain MENTALLY AGILE enough to be able to enjoy our healthy independence?

We, as consumers, are becoming more health-conscious when it comes to maintaining a healthy diet for our BODIES, but will that be good enough to sustain a HEALTHY BRAIN?

There is such a thing as BRAIN FOOD. Hydration is the key that will help maintain a healthy brain, and it is recommended that we drink as much as 2-4 litres of water a day. The brain is made up of 90% water, and when we become dehydrated, our minds can become sluggish, we can go into auto-pilot mode, and your inner child starts to make some bad choices.

Chances are when you are feeling thirsty, you are already dehydrated.

Drinking water as soon as I wake up in the morning has become a morning ritual for me because unless I have a drink during the night, I am depriving my body and mind of water for a good few hours while I am asleep.

Do you know what foods ARE good for your BODY and BRAIN?
Most supermarket chains advertise healthy options, but in our experience, the healthy options are not that healthy for us.

Just because it's gluten-free, doesn't mean that it's healthy!

A lot of the gluten free products you might find will have sugar, sweeteners and vegetable oils, which are all very inflammatory and should be avoided.

In my opinion, if it comes in a bag, a packet, a box or a tin, then you should have a look at the ingredients and question whether it really is any good for you.

Another general rule, if you have seen it on a TV advert, then it's probably not as healthy as they make it out to be. You don't see many adverts for fruits and vegetables, do you?

There are so many cereal bars and so-called "healthy", low-fat, low-calorie products out these days and, with a massive media drive to promote them, it's very understandable why we get sucked into thinking that these are good for us.

Nothing could be further from the truth. There is probably very little goodness in any of them whatsoever.

Remember – just eat real food. This is what is best for your body, for your health, your energy and your waistline.

Quite often, a lot of the marketed "healthy" products are actually higher in calories, salt, sugar and bad fats.

Remember, it's not the saturated fats that are bad for you; it's the 'Trans fats' that are in processed foods so don't eat the packaged stuff even if it's marketed as "healthy".

Even the 'low-fat, low-calorie' kinds are often worse than the 'full-fat, original' versions, look at yoghurts for instance. Tonnes of low-fat options but loaded with sugar and sweeteners. We are far better taking the full-fat options such as real butter, full-fat yoghurt and cream.

Remember, it's not really the calories that you should be concerned about; it's the sugar and carbs, and often the trans fats.

Artificial trans fats are formed when cooking oil goes through a process called hydrogenation, which makes the oil solidify (known as hardening). The oil is then used in the cooking of some processed food.

Artificial trans fats can be found in some processed foods such as biscuits and cakes, where they are sometimes used to help give products a longer shelf life.

Diet drinks and diet foods are just processed versions of the original products, which are essentially just as bad so don't assume that because you chose the 'light' option that this will be better for your health or your weight.

Food companies have had an absolute field day since the low-fat boom, convincing us that we should eat their low-calorie and low-fat processed products and as a result, we are getting sicker and fatter and even more confused as to why.

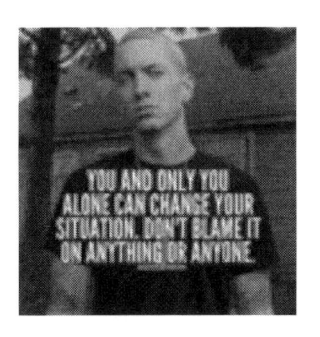

When it comes to making the right choices for food:
- Eat fresh products
- Pre-prepare your week's food (in advance)
- Plan a weekly menu
- Only shop for what is on your list
- Avoid the low-fat and healthy labels

Let's examine the components that our foods comprise.

Protein

Protein is made up of amino acids, which are the building blocks for your muscles, therefore, are essential to the body.

They are essential, meaning that we have to get them from food.
Protein is crucial for refuelling and repairing your muscles and your cells.

Your protein intake should probably always stay the same, whereas your fat and carb intake can be changed according to your results and your activity levels.

Proteins are the important ingredients in the elasticity of the brain (its ability to generate new neural pathways) because the glia (the web that connects neurones together) is entirely made up of proteins.

Carbohydrates

Every day, our bodies need fuel to survive and function properly.

That fuel is made up of protein, carbs and fats, and let's not forget water.

Despite what we are led to believe, carbs are not the most important macro nutrient – this is another big myth that is robbing us of a healthy fit body and one that is costing us money on health care in the long run as well.

In fact, unlike protein and fat, carbs are actually the only macronutrient that isn't essential, meaning we don't actually need to consume carbs whatsoever.

This might seem controversial, especially for those of us who were taught that we NEED carbs as energy if we are partaking in exercise.

It isn't necessary to eat carbs, and it certainly isn't vital that we eat anywhere near as many as we do or as we are advised.

Think about it, back in the caveman days, we hadn't had access to all of the carbs and sugar-based products that we have today, nor all the low-fat and low-calorie stuff.

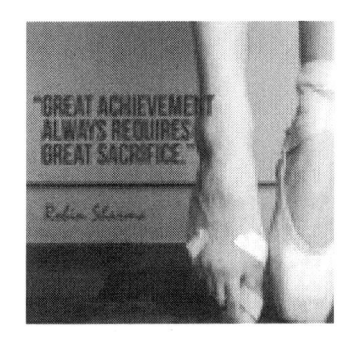

Our diets mainly consisted of full-fat, medium protein and a slight amount of carbs and sugar from seasonal fruits.

We ate these carbs to fatten us up so that we could survive the winter months when food would be hard to come by. It was also a strategy adopted by most European countries after the last world war when food was very scarce.

Does this mean that we should avoid carbs altogether? No, not unless you wanted to, which wouldn't do you any harm, but all I am saying is that we really don't need to eat as many as we currently do and again nowhere near as many as we are now advised.

Vegetables and fruits still contain carbohydrates – these are perfectly fine.

Vegetables can be eaten in unlimited quantities and are an excellent source of vitamins, minerals, and antioxidants. They are full of phytonutrients, which are anti-inflammatory. Veggies are also full of fibre.

Low-sugar fruits, in small quantities, are also a good source of vitamins and minerals and antioxidants, such as blueberries, kiwis, etc.

Fats

Fat, despite what we have been told, is not bad for us.

Fat is essential for the brain and the body.

Fat is also vital for hormone and cell production.

Low dietary fat intake has been shown to have a reduction in brain function and linked with behavioural problems, memory function, depression, anxiety and also Alzheimer's.

Back in the caveman days, our diets would have consisted of around 75% fat which is a far cry from what we are advised that it should be today, which is around 20%.

There is no need to fear healthy fat unless it's trans fats in processed and packaged foods. Always read the label!

Brain foods

Foods that are good for the brain are those that are high in natural fats such as wild salmon and deep water fish that are high in Omega-3.

According to Steven Pratt (MD of Superfoods), we can fight off the ageing brain if we can add into our diet these following foods:

- Blueberries or *brainberries* are high in antioxidants and are said to stave off Alzheimer's and dementia.
- Nuts and seeds (except peanuts or any roasted or salted) contain natural essential fats and are a good source of vitamin E, which has been proven to maintain the cognitive function of the brain, especially as we age.
- Avocados are just as good as blueberries, plus they contain natural fats that help promote a healthy blood flow and reduce cholesterol. Maintaining a healthy blood

flow to the brain is essential as it needs a constant supply to keep it functioning.
- Wild Salmon and any oily fish such as mackerel, sardines and pilchards because they are high in Omega-3 oils and other anti-inflammatory substances, which are necessary for generating new brain cells.
- Whole Grains such as oats can also contain Omega-3, fibre and vitamin E. We recommend the gluten-free option that is now available in most supermarkets.
- Beans, black beans and lentils are known to stabilise blood sugar levels in the body while providing the brain with its preferred fuel (glucose). The brain lacks fuel stores and requires a continuous supply of glucose. It consumes about 120g per day.
- Pomegranate Juice: the sugar-free and natural version is the most potent in antioxidants because it contains almost every antioxidant.
- Green Tea has a superb effect on the body, including antitoxins, and together with other fruit teas (ginger and honey), they have other benefits that keep the brain from free radicals that damage cell rejuvenation and contribute to ageing.
- Dark Chocolate, although it contains some antioxidants, it also releases endorphins which make you feel good. Caution: it also contains caffeine and some sugars. We recommend the 70%+ of cocoa in moderation.

We also recommend using coconut oils for cooking too as this is one of the few oils that doesn't change its composition when heated up. You may have to reduce the heat as you cook with it but it is superb for your body and brain, again keeping them free of free radicals.

Finally, water is the source of life or at least where our brains are concerned. Dehydration will cause a loss of brain function because the brain is made up of 75% water. It is essential that you get at least 2-4 litres of water into your body because only a small percentage of it will reach your brain.

For further information and recipe ideas, check out our LBP cookbooks via our website www.theleanbodyproject.co.uk

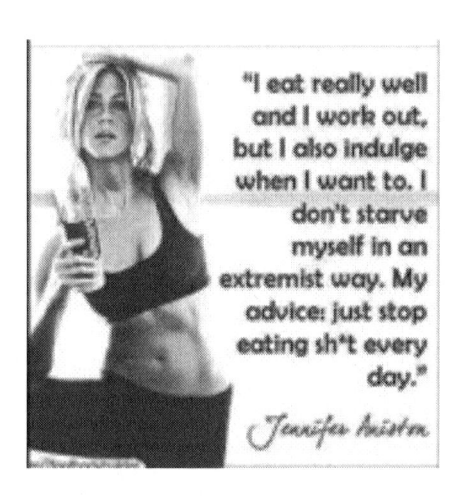

> "I eat really well and I work out, but I also indulge when I want to. I don't starve myself in an extremist way. My advice: just stop eating sh*t every day."
>
> *Jennifer Aniston*

Sleep

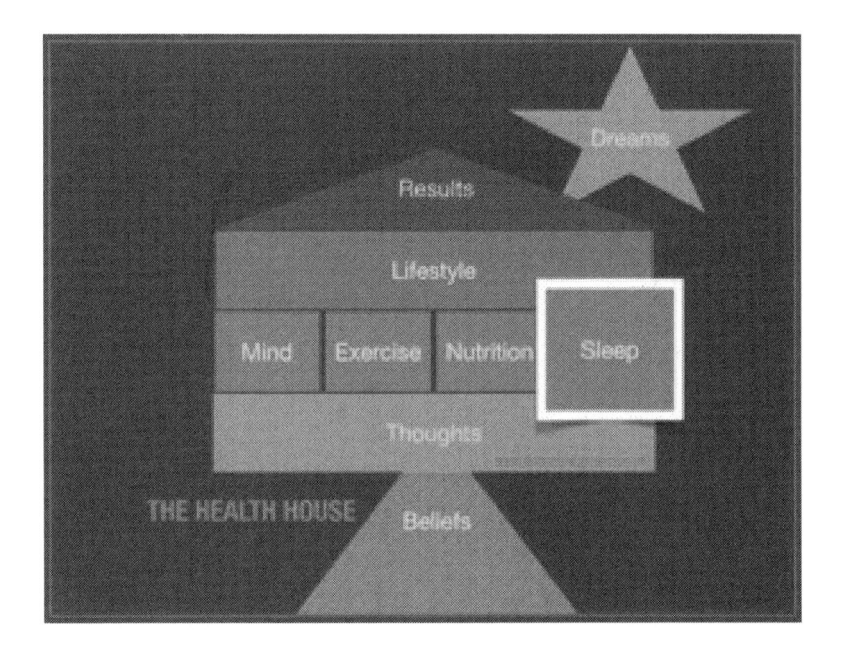

SLEEP (Rest) YOURSELF THINNER!

One of the most underrated aspects of the FAT LOSS process is that of rest and sleep, according to the National Sleep Foundation.

In fact, recent studies by the University of Chicago Medical Centre have demonstrated that lack of QUALITY rest and sleep actually mess up your hormone levels (Cortisol) and affect metabolism, which directly impacts on your appetite making you want to eat.

A recent study pointed to the possible causes of DIABETES being insulin sensitivity and glucose reduction. The results showed that the body reacts negatively to the lack of sleep which makes it more sensitive to insulin, which is a precursor to diabetes.

Alternatively, those of us that want to add lean muscle also underestimate the power of rest days and a good night's sleep. It seems that our bodies need to recuperate to build and repair itself.

When it comes to health, we tend to highlight VISCERAL FAT as active fat that is stored within the abdominal cavity (stomach) and is, therefore, collected around a number of vital internal organs such as the liver, pancreas and intestines.

In short, if your body is constantly on the go, and your hormone levels are out of sync, then it is unlikely that you will be a FAT BURNING machine.

It needs to rest after exercise so that it can replenish its stores in preparation for the next bout of activity.

Depending on which research you read, the recommendations are anywhere from 4-9 hours of sleep per day and at least 2-3 days in every 7 of rest.

Our opinion is that everybody is different and therefore one size cannot fit all, especially when it comes to sleep. Listen to your body and if you feel tired, then SLEEP and if your performance is not where it should be, then REST. You will often find that a good rest day can often improve performance because you have more energy.

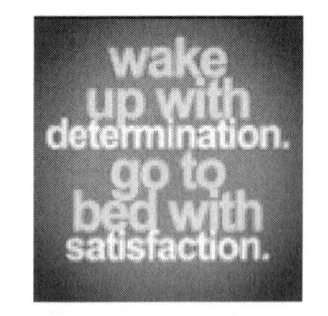

wake up with determination. go to bed with satisfaction.

SLEEP is the unsung hero of FAT LOSS, and REST is the essential ingredient for your BEST PERFORMANCE.

It's good for your mind as well as your body because it is your 'MASTER GLAND'. Remember, that controls the hormone levels in your body!

Here are a few things that prevent you from sleeping:

- Alcohol: although it seems that it is a good aid to help you drift off, the reality is that as the alcohol is broken down in your body, it has the opposite effect and can frequently wake you up. Even though you initially fall into a deeper sleep, your temperature regulator kicks in as your body temperature increases.
- High-protein supper: although we at LBP have a high-protein nutrition program, it is not recommended to eat a protein-packed meal before you go to sleep. As your body is breaking down the nutrients, it is also encouraging your brain to create energy-booting neurochemicals which will make it hard to initiate sleep.
- Using electronic devices just before going to bed. It appears that the false light triggers something in our brains and stimulates it rather than relaxing it. Using your phone or tablet while in bed will make getting off to sleep more difficult, so put a curfew on it at least an hour before.
- Sometimes, the smallest of lights can creep through our eyelids and keep us awake. Try covering the alarm clock and stand-by lights in your bedroom. Install blackout blinds and/or heavy curtains so that you can maximise your sleep.

According to Prof Colin Smith of the University of Surrey, in a recent study those who had less than 6-hour sleep per night, had a 90% risk of being obese than those who had 7-8 hours of sleep. Sleep deprived people feel hungrier and tend to eat higher calorie meals than those who get enough rest.

The hormone imbalance due to lack of sleep produces more 'ghrelin' (hunger hormone) coupled with a reduction of leptin, which tells the body when it's full, is a disastrous combination when you are trying to lose weight.

Here are some tips on how to stay asleep or nod off again after waking:

- How dark can you make your bedroom? It seems that darkness triggers our natural sleeping hormone, 'melatonin', which promotes a restful night's sleep. Thick or black out curtains, blinds and, although it's a bit of a passion killer, you may consider a sleep mask.
- Sleepy tea: Clipper easy sleep tea bags are a natural remedy for instigating sleep. Perfect for a nightcap before heading to bed. It contains herbs that are well-known for relaxing the body, including valerian, chamomile and cinnamon.
- If you are one of those people that regularly gets up in the night to use the toilet, then you may want to consider exactly when you last have a drink before you go to bed. Also, try going to the loo before you brush your teeth and again after you have undressed yourself but before you actually get into bed. This technique is called double voiding and it ensures that the bladder is completely empty, which could help you sleep undisturbed.
- How old is your mattress? If you constantly toss and turn in your sleep trying to find a comfy position, then you may either have the wrong mattress for you or it may need updating. The rule of thumb is that we should change our mattress every 10 years or so.
- Maintaining a cool temperature in your bedroom will help you get a good night's sleep. Apparently, your body needs to cool down to 18-20C to induce sleep.

So let's say that you have dropped off to sleep but have woken up for whatever reason and are now struggling to get back to sleep, and you keep checking the alarm clock every hour.

If you are struggling to get back to sleep once you have woken up, then you might want to try this 'Jedi' mind trick on yourself.

When your brain has started to wake up, you begin what the Buddhists call 'The Monkey Chatter' because of the way a monkey can incessantly talk and distract you. They compare it to having a monkey in your head that just won't shut up. They also say that to quieten the monkey you have to give it a task to do. Focus on your breaths and count them but also slow them down if you can.

I use a slightly different technique that I call 'The Yawn' method. So called because a yawn is one of the most infectious things that can happen in a room full of people. As soon as one person does it, you can guarantee that someone else will also follow soon afterwards.

Whatever your "monkey" is chattering about, I want you to slow it right down as if being said by someone that is very tired and in the middle of a yawn too. You see, your brain will also begin to slow down as you yawn and slowly drift back off to sleep. Repeat if necessary where you are struggling to quieten your mind.

One final thing on the subject of sleep and how to obtain a good night's sleep if you are one of those that just can't stop your brain from working and think about the things that you have to do.

I suggest that you get yourself a pad and a pen or pencil. Place them by the side of your bed, so that when you awake in the night with a thought of the things that you need to do, just write them down on the pad. It seems that once we have written something down that we want to remember, we may subconsciously STOP thinking about it.

Try reading an old-fashioned book, with real pages and written text. The reason for reading a physical book is that, unlike the electronic counterparts, it has no backlight, which, as we know, stimulates the active part of the brain.

Reading a book not only helps you to learn – and should be part of your daily schedule – but it also tires your eyes out. The muscles in the eyes become tired over time, and that tricks the brain into thinking that it is ready to go to sleep – unless you find a magnificent book that you are unable to put down and then you can stay awake for hours, gripped in the story.

Lavender plants are also said to promote sleep because of their natural relaxing properties. Try putting one of these in your bedroom, providing that you don't have any allergies.

Summary

- Remember that when it comes to your happiness, your thoughts and your life, you have the ability to choose how it all pans out. It is your movie and if you don't like where you are in life, change the channel and become the main character.

- Remove some of those subconscious decisions that your inner child might make about what you eat, when you exercise and how your day is going to go. Plan your meals weekly and shop accordingly. Also, join a fitness community so that you'll have the support of like-minded people that will be there to support you when you most need it.

- You CANNOT out-train a bad diet! Although exercise will accelerate your fat loss when combined with a healthy nutrition plan, it is possible to get to the shape that you want purely with the right nutritional plan.

- The benefits of exercise to our health is unprecedented for as little as 10 minutes of high-intensity training or 30-40 minutes of light to moderate exercise. It doesn't matter what you do, just do something and don't wait until a Monday to start, just get moving today.

- Having the right nutritional plan that works for you is critical because there are lots of diets and weekly fads that are all out there to make money from you. Eating cleanly, with fresh food that is free from added sugars and preservatives, etc., will make the biggest difference to the quality of your life. Last but not least, make sure you drink plenty of water (2-4 litres per day).

- Sleep is the unsung hero of fat loss and a healthier you. The quality of sleep, regardless of how much your body and mind needs, will differ from person to person. There is no such thing as 'one size fits all' when it comes to sleep. Quality over quantity.

Chapter 5
Lifestyle

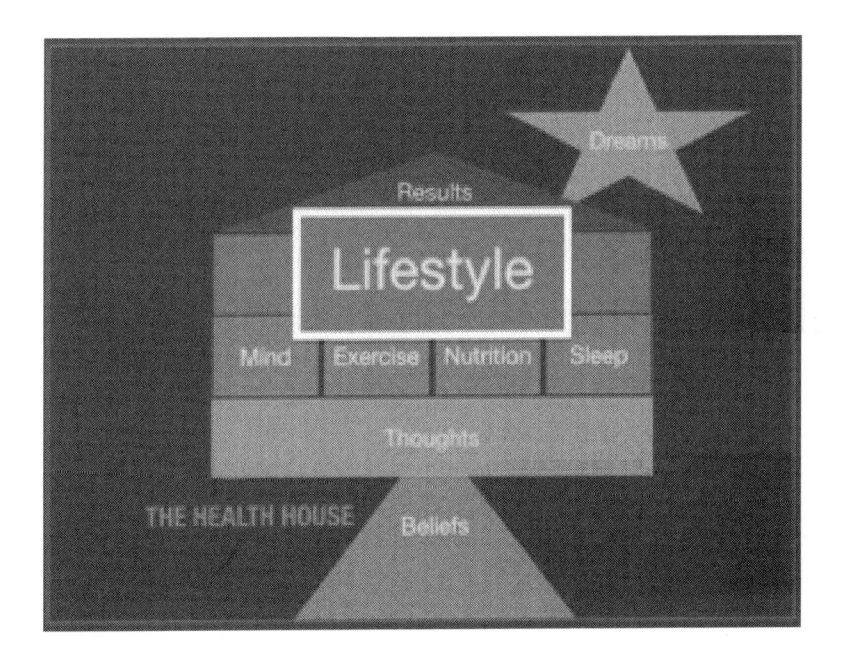

What does your lifestyle say about you?

Are you constantly in a rush and always on the last minute, or do you start something with plenty of energy only to lose interest and focus?

We don't necessarily think about all those conscious and subconscious decisions that we make on a daily basis because most of them have become HABITS.

Many of us don't STOP to think about the everyday choices that are available to us and, instead, surrender ourselves to the habitual decisions of what to eat, how we behave and ultimately the RESULTS that we get.

I genuinely believe in the sincerity of intention when people make their New Year's resolutions, but what is the one thing that always remains the same?

Answer: YOU.

People are motivated either TOWARDS or AWAY from their goals, depending on the accumulation of their daily choices.

STOP and ask yourself, 'Is what I am doing adding to or subtracting from my goals?'

Most people don't realise that each time that you start to do something and don't complete it, it is actually subconsciously destroying your self-confidence!

Make this year the year that you SHOW UP and be the VERY BEST VERSION of yourself, each and every day in 2017! Make decisions that your future self in 2018 will thank you for.

First, ensure that you check whether your New Year's resolution is worth the price that you MUST PAY to get it.

Next, ask yourself how serious you are on a scale of 1-10, and if you are anything less than a 10, then you aren't serious enough to get what you want.

Detox your life! If you are really decisive about achieving your goal, then get rid of all the things that will get in your way – this may include a circle of your friends!

Choose one major thing to focus on because if you try and do too much at the same time, you run the risk of becoming overwhelmed, and this will result in failure.

ONLY when your lifestyle reflects the desire to become who you need to become to get what you want out of life does the magic begin to happen.

Top tip: 'Life begins at the end of your comfort zone.' ~ Neale Walsh

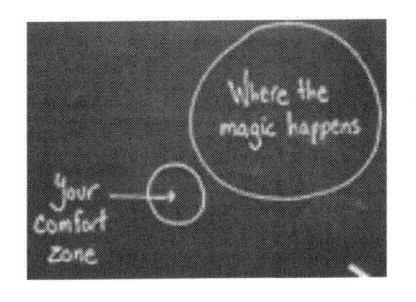

It's that imaginary boundary that we all have, and we tend to get very anxious when we come to the edge of it.

It's like believing that the earth is flat and if we sail past the coast of South Africa, we will fall into an eternal abyss, never to be heard of again.

'Ships are only safe in the harbour, but that is not what they were made for.' ~ William G.T. Shed.

Our comfort zone seems to be at the edge of our daily habits. You know, those things that we do every day without having to engage our brain too much. Those things that you do now just because you have always done them and even though they may not bear any relevance to your life today, you continue to do them because they are Ingrained Habitual Behaviours (IHB).

Your amazing brain is able to create brand new synapses and neural pathways instantly if you harness the power of your thoughts. Similar to walking through the long grass during a country walk: you can barely make out the path, but there is a new pathway; if you look hard enough, you can almost make one out.

The more that you walk through that path, the more evident it will become, until you have walked it ten or twenty times and you can see the well-trodden path as plain as day.

This is a simple way of describing how habits are formed in our mind. The reason that we develop habits is that we have so much information that we have to contend with during the day. If we were to attempt to concentrate on every bit of information, then we would literally end up in a straitjacket.

Instead, our brains 'chunk up' information and store it in the back of our long-term memory (subconscious mind) so that we are able to perform a task without having to think about it, such as driving a car.

If you think back to when you were taking driving lessons, you had to concentrate on new skills like indicating, looking in the mirror, steering, releasing the clutch and pressing the accelerator at the same time. It took time for you to build on them before they became second nature. If you don't drive, you can use your imagination regarding the complexity of driving a car while simultaneously reading the road.

What do your daily habits say about you? Which ones are stopping you from achieving your dreams? What thing would make the biggest difference to your lifestyle if you just stopped doing it?

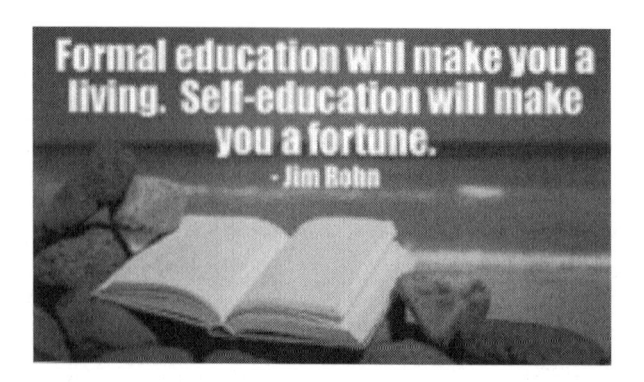

> **Formal education will make you a living. Self-education will make you a fortune.**
> - Jim Rohn

Let's take a look at your morning routine right now. List all the things that you do from the moment that you open your eyes to the time that you leave for work.

What time do you wake up?
How many times do you press snooze?
What is the first thing that you do when you get out of bed?
How much time do you spend watching TV?
What do you eat for breakfast?
What do you drink?
What do you say to yourself while getting ready in the morning?
Do you take your lunch with you?
How much time do you invest in developing yourself each day?
Do you take the chance to say 'I love you' to your loved ones?

How many of you believe that you are NOT a morning person? Or that you are unable to function without your second cup of coffee or tea?

Really? Are you actually telling me that you are physically unable to perform and that if your kettle suddenly blew up, then you would have to call in to say to your boss, 'Sorry boss, I can't come in today because my kettle is broken.'?

Of course, you wouldn't because you know how ridiculous that would sound and, furthermore, if you think that the world will end because you have run out of coffee or tea, then you may have a caffeine addiction.

The crux of the matter is that if you tell yourself that you are not a morning person, then remember that your subconscious mind (inner child) will agree with you until you genuinely believe that you are unable to function in the morning.

Hundreds of years ago before the introduction of mainstream electricity, we lived by candlelight and awoke with nature. The sunrise would provide the natural light for which to work by, and the sound of the cockerel would act as nature's alarm clock.

The working day started as early as 5 am for some people, and as long as there was daylight, then there was work to be done. Thank goodness for electricity, modern technology and civilised working hours!

Do you jump out of bed at the last minute, hugging that pillow and milking each second until you have to get up, then rush around like an idiot, skip breakfast and wake up on the journey to work only to realise that you still have your PJ's on?

Whatever your routine, I guarantee that 99% of it will be an ingrained habitual behaviour. If you are one of those who keeps telling yourself and others that you don't have enough time in your day to exercise or prepare food or read or any of the other things that you tell yourself in your story, then this chapter is definitely for you.

An excellent resource on this is 'Miracle Morning' by Hal Elrod. The book encapsulates what my morning routine used to be and, if anything, helped me to make it more efficient.

Your daily routine says a lot about your attitude towards the day and life, in general. Let me explain.
'What does it matter what time I wake up in the morning?', I hear you say. Well, let me give you an overview of my typical day before 9 am.

5:45 am - wake up, get dressed and feed the dog.
6:00 - mindset statements, read a chapter of a book while drinking green tea, after taking Omega-3 fish oil capsules and vitamin C, washed down with 1/2 litre filtered water.
7:00 - spin class
7:30 - weights session
8:30 - home for a shower, breakfast, prepare today's meals-to-go and check some emails.

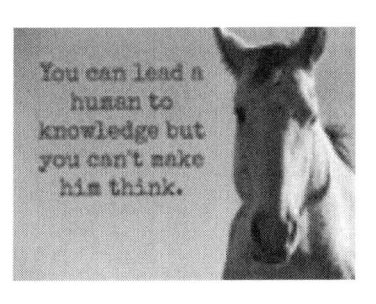

Introducing 'Parkinson's Time' law:

'Work expands to fill the time that it is allotted.'

This means that whatever time we allow to complete a task, that said time will actually take us to do it. This usually works by leaving it until the last minute and then working twice as hard to complete it! However, it also works if you allow some 20-30 minutes a day to complete a task too.

Writing a book, for example. If you committed to writing just one blog post a day at 5 or 6 am, then you would soon have enough content for your book, certainly within a few months anyway.

Before you even say to yourself, 'Oh, I need at least 10 hours of sleep each night,' I want you to think about what message that gives to your subconscious mind! Each person will require a different amount of time to rest, and again, there is no one-size-fits-all.

It is also why people always start their new "healthy habits" on a Monday! If you are really serious about it, then why would you wait until Monday, why wouldn't you start immediately? This is because most people want a blowout during the weekend and wrongly believe that they deserve to relax and go into Friday on auto pilot. Not if you are serious about this stuff!

It does matter what time you get up because if you always do things at the last minute, rushing around, it shows that you are generally unprepared and you seldom put in any research but, instead, prefer to take unnecessary risks.

Type 1: The chances are you will be one of those people that shop for their lunch at lunch time and, each evening, will decide what they are going to eat for their evening meal. The only challenge in doing this is that if you rely on what you FANCY to eat, then there is the likelihood of you choosing something unhealthy.

If you have ever been shopping when you are starving and come out of the supermarket with more than you needed or planned, then you know what I mean.

If you have planned your meals in advance and pre-prepared them at least, you take away the emotion from the equation. But if you rely on your emotions to make decisions about what you may or may not want for your evening meals, then you'll also rely on the emotions of the day too.

Let's imagine that you have had a bad day all round and you have been reprimanded at work. You may be forgiven for feeling a little upset and then throw into the mix your journey home that takes 2 hours longer than it should.

What might be the first thing you do when you walk into your house? What is your crux? What is the thing that you do, the place that you go to when you are feeling down or depressed? Is it that faithful glass of wine, beer, a chocolate bar, a cake? What are the chances of you attending the gym or fitness class at this point?

Now throw into the mix the decision of what you are going to eat for your evening meal. What do you think the chances are of it being healthy or will it be the faithful takeaway service or simply a ready meal?

Type 2: Have you ever woken up just before the alarm or do you jump out of bed as soon as it goes off? Then you are one of the minority few that attack the day with vigour, you know what you want and how to get it.

You are more likely to plan your meals and shop according to your planned menu. You will be able to take away the emotion from the decision because the decision has already been made, and you know what you are having for your meal. It is likely to be healthy, and you stand a better chance of sticking to your plan. Preparation is key for you.

Type 3: If you press the snooze button several times before you even think about lifting your head from the pillow, this suggests that you would rather hibernate in your bed and most probably lack energy and determination in life.

You probably still live at home with your parents or live with someone who makes all these decisions for you while you play Xbox games with your mates.

- Top tip: Move your alarm clock away from your bedroom so that you have to get out of bed to turn it off. You will be more likely to get up without a snooze!

- Go brush your teeth and maybe use some mouthwash. Science has proven that just refreshing your mouth will increase your waking consciousness.

- Have at least a half-litre of water. Science shows that we dehydrate during the night as we sleep, and after 8 hours or so of water deprivation, your brain will need to hydrate.

- Some say affirmations (feel-good statements about themselves) each morning in the mirror or at least out loud. Some pray, some use the time to read their Bible while others just use the time to expand their mind. Whatever you choose to do, please DO IT consistently.

- What do you watch or listen to in the morning? Ask yourself if it is positive or negative. If you are constantly taking in negative information, guess what that is going to do to your mindset. Change the channel or turn it off and try our 30-day challenge.

- Exercise at least 20 minutes a day at a high intensity (HIT) is proven to not only burn fat and start your metabolism, so it continues throughout the day, but it also has huge benefits to your brain by increasing the blood flow and oxygen, which are essential to brain function.

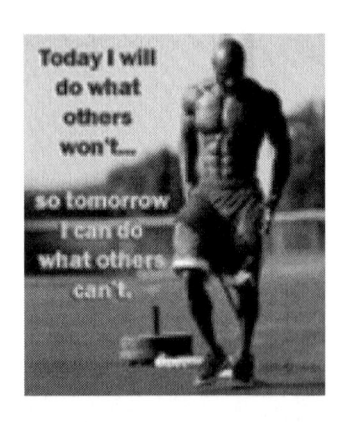

It only takes between 3 to 28 days to break a habit and install a new one in your brain.

What one thing do you know that if you just stopped doing today would absolutely make a significant difference to the quality of your life?

Equally, what one thing do you instinctively know that if you started to do right now, would make the biggest positive difference to your life immediately?

On the left-hand side of the box below, make a list of all the barriers that prevent you from achieving your goals. On the right, make a list of the things that will enable your success.

Once you have a list, notice how many are in your control and how many are out of your control? Now strike through all the things that are out of your control.

You should be left with a list of barriers and a list of enablers that are in your control and that you can do something about. There isn't much point in worrying about those things that you cannot control, so let's control the controllable.

Barriers	Enablers

Of the things on the list, how many can you deal with immediately and you may have just been putting them off? If the reasons for the postponement are genuine, then leave them on there, and we will address them next.

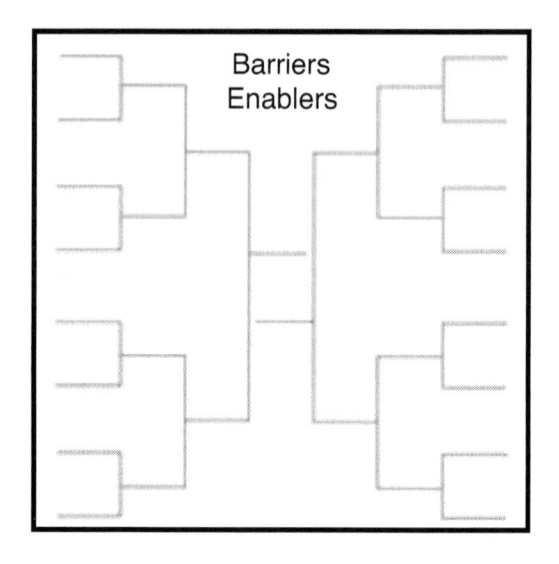

Barriers
Enablers

If you are a sports fan, you will probably recognise the image above because it is similar to the one used for sports tournaments. Generally, each horizontal line on the outside left would have 8 different team/player names on and same on the right-hand side. The winner of the two teams that play each other goes through to the next round, and they play with the winners of the other matches until you have only two teams left in the final.

Populate this in terms of priority starting with your Barriers and your Enablers and rank them regarding their priority. Put those with the highest priority through to the next round and continue until the process is complete and you have 1 Barrier and 1 Enabler left.

These are what you should address as a matter of priority. There will be a cost involved as there is in most cases, and following on from your previous exercise, you will have a pretty good understanding of what that cost will be.

There will be a cost regarding:
- Time
- Effort
- Money
- Sweat
- Sacrifice

What are you willing to sacrifice to achieve your goals? Now that you know the cost involved, you may decide that the price is just TOO HIGH. In which case, choose a different goal.

Time is an objective cost. I mean you might have to spend a minimum amount of time preparing your food on a weekend, 30 minutes to an hour a day exercising, plus travel to and from your fitness class or gym. When you add all this time up it will be a considerable amount of not only from your week but also from your weekend too. If you add into that the extra time that you will need to invest in developing yourself, it may well eat into the evenings when you would normally watch your favourite soaps.

All this could possibly take time away from your family or your business or hobbies too. It may well be that the timing isn't quite right for you. I mean if you are experiencing a 'Significant Emotional Experience' in your life right now, it will either work for you or against you.

The expenditure of effort will continue to be the biggest spend that you have because preparing food and working out meal plans, exercise routines and self-development, all require effort. And the more work you put into something, the more rewarding the outcome and generally more self-gratifying. Speaking from experience, getting up on those cold dark winter mornings to exercise requires a lot of discipline but even more effort.

The financial cost might mean that you have to allow a monthly health club subscription, an extra budget for your grocery shopping, clothes, equipment and professional support. There will be a monetary cost to you and your family, and you have to ask yourself if the price is worth paying.

Not to be confused with effort, but you will have to pay in sweat and perspiration. There will be times when your mind will tell you to give up because it can't take any more. Here is a fact from the military: when your mind has had enough, your body has still got another 40% to give you!

We have already briefly mentioned some of the sacrifices that you might have to make to get what you want. You will definitely have to sacrifice sugar, alcohol, bread, pasta, pastries and caffeine to become really lean. This is because they either bloat you up, clog you up, dehydrate you and make you store excess water.

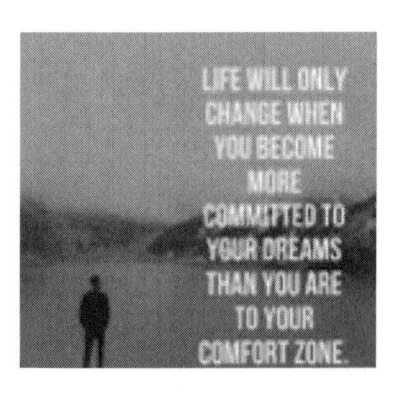

LIFE WILL ONLY CHANGE WHEN YOU BECOME MORE COMMITTED TO YOUR DREAMS THAN YOU ARE TO YOUR COMFORT ZONE.

You may have to sacrifice time with your friends socialising until you get your body into the shape that you are happy with.

Whatever you choose to do, there is a price to pay, and this particular store, the store of life, doesn't give discounts or shortcuts. It requires that you pay in full first before you can achieve your desired goal.

Show up each day and be the very best version of you that you can be.

I've heard so many people say the phrase 'show up' but what does it really mean? You have to be present at the HIT class and you have to turn up to support your friends and family, right?

My take on this phrase is simple, it is not enough for you to just be present, it is not enough for you to just go through the motions and it is certainly not enough to just make a half-hearted attempt at making healthy food choices.

In my mind, you either choose TO or choose NOT to, which is it?

Showing up is throwing yourself into every situation and immersing yourself in your own healthy world, entirely dedicated, and demonstrating it with every choice that you make throughout the day.

Whether you are supporting someone else on social media, planning your week's menu, eating out with friends at social gatherings, joining in a fitness class, give it everything that you have and don't leave anything in the tank.

Successful people, show up each and every day of their lives which is what makes them successful. They don't falter at the first sign of difficulty but instead choose to find a workaround. It is this level of determination that will get you the life that you so much desire and deserve.

It is my sincere wish that you attain the health, shape and body that you so much want in your life, you deserve it and don't let anyone tell you otherwise.

Detox your life

At this point, I will make two profound axioms:

1. You are where you are in your life due to the accretion of the choices that you have made on a daily basis.
2. 'You are the accumulation of the 5 people, whom you spend the most time with.' ~ Jim Rohn

During the 2012 Olympic games in London, one particular sport dominated the headlines for Team GB: cycling. A now Sir David Brailsford who had coached the team to success had reportedly attributed their success to the accumulation of marginal gains.

They were said to use a podium principle which combined their strategy, their performance and continuous improvement. 'We were precise about food preparation. We brought our own mattresses and pillows so our athletes could sleep in the same posture every night. We searched for small improvements everywhere and found countless opportunities. Taken together, we felt they gave us a competitive advantage.'

In principle, it shares many similarities with Darren Hardy's 'compound effect'. In which the smallest positive change in your life might seem only insignificant in the multitude of choices that you make on a daily basis. Over a time period of a year, however, it will have a significant effect on your life.

Take breakfast for example, if you only committed to having a healthy 'clean' breakfast for 1 year, the changes will not be evident at first, and yet, after 12 months, you may feel a whole lot better and lose a few pounds in the process.

Another and perhaps a more significant example would be to reduce your sugar intake. Let's say that you take two spoons full of sugar in your coffee. Now cutting your intake by one spoon will not make a huge difference in the first week, but over a few months, you will have reduced your intake by half.

It is the accumulation of those small and somewhat insignificant choices that will either make or break you. The smallest choices that you make now regarding your food, exercise and mindset will make a huge difference to you in a few months.

Would you have made any different choices this week, now that you know?

> Write down the choices that you have made in the past week that you wish you could change:

Now write down the 5 people whom you spend the most time with.

> The names of the 5 people that I spend the most time with are:
>
> 1.
>
> 2.
>
> 3.
>
> 4.
>
> 5.

Think for a moment about some of those people and their values, traits, attitudes, beliefs and behaviours. Do you like everything about them or are there parts of their personality that you don't particularly like?

One of the many things that I had picked up at university was to spend time with those in the year above me because they had been where I was and experienced what lay in store for me over the coming year. The more time I spent with them, the more I learned and started to get ahead.

If you want to get ahead in life, then seek out those like-minded people. Those that are either going through the same journey as you or are further down the road than you regarding fitness. I guarantee that you will instinctively start to raise your game.

Now that you know this nugget of information, would you choose a different set of people?

For you to get healthier and fitter, you may have to be prepared to detox your life not only from the toxins that you put into your body but also from the environment in which you spend the most time. Are you prepared to cut some of those people out of your life while you are getting healthy?

If your friends are making you fat, then you should choose some different friends until you have the body that you want and you are where you want to be in life. Detoxing your life means every part of your life, and not just your diet, for a few weeks because being healthy is a lifestyle choice.

Here are 8 toxic people that you should leave out of your life:

1. Those who spread negativity
2. Those who criticise you all the time
3. Those who waste your time
4. Those who are jealous
5. Those who play the victim
6. Those who don't care
7. Those who are self-centred

8. Those who keep disappointing you

Make a line in the sand and be brutal! Stand up for yourself and stop tolerating these people. There is an old saying 'you get what you tolerate,' and it refers to letting people's behaviour just slide because you are too polite.

It is your life, and you are the main character in this movie of your life. But if you are letting other people bring you down and you are spending your life trying to please those around you, then you are only ever going to be a supporting actor in your movie because if you are not living your dreams and aspirations, then you will end up living some else's. Trust me when I say that there are plenty of people out there that would gladly have you do that.

Until you are strong enough to truly believe in you and that you are sufficient, you should cut yourself some slack.

If they are real friends, then they will understand while you get yourself together. If they are not, then do you really want them in your life?

Summary

- What habits do you have on a daily basis that you know if you just stopped them immediately, they would have a significant impact on your health? Change just one habit at a time and remember that it only takes between 3 to 28 days to reprogram your Ingrained Habitual Behaviours (IHB).

- Work out the price of your new healthy life and decide whether it is worth paying and commit to how far you are willing to go to get this new lifestyle. Remember that you will pay in full, and there is no discount at the store of life.

- Show up every day, once you have committed to action, give it everything that you have got and leave nothing in the tank. Be the very best version of you that you can be so that you do everything to the very best of your ability, no excuses.

- Be prepared to detox your life. What areas of your life need a spring clean right now? What's holding you back? What resources do you need and where can you go to find them?

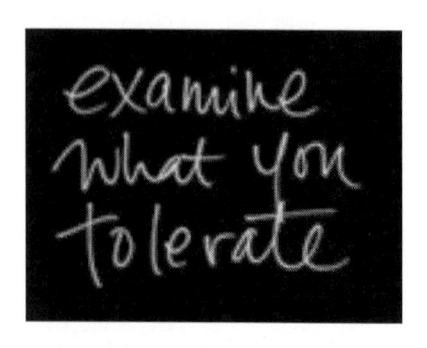

> *examine what you tolerate*

Chapter 6
Dreams

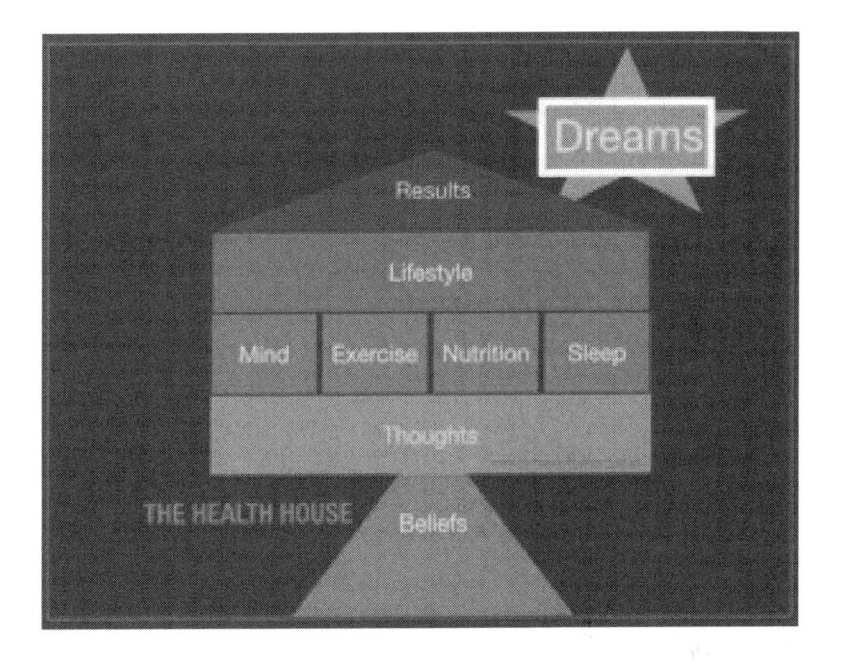

Dreams are those wonderful things that happen when we allow our minds to wander and roam through the meadows of our imagination.

A little bit of science

The same part of the brain that is responsible for making the decision to do something is the same part of the brain that performs the action, the prefrontal cortex, where decisions are made and acted upon according to studies from a university in Iowa.

'Cognitive control and value-based decision-making tasks appear to depend on different brain regions within the prefrontal cortex,' says Jan Glascher in Time magazine, 2012.

The prefrontal cortex is the same part of the brain that steers us towards the things that we want, and it is also the same part that keeps us from overindulging too. When shopping in supermarkets, people generally go armed with a list of items that they need.

On the way, round the supermarket, we are bombarded with tempting items that we might just fancy. The executive decision process is the very thing that can either help us to stay on track and focused or prevent us from achieving.

In an article published in Scientific American by John Pearson, Michael Platt on August 5, 2008. They proposed that the rationale for this is that the decision making was dependent on neural plasticity which is the brain's ability to create new thought pathways.

In doing so, the brain 'eavesdrops' on all the other potential thoughts that we at LBP call 'interference'. Just as a TV can produce a weak signal due to inclement weather, the brain can also make a poor executive decision due to the interfering mind chatter.

If it is indeed the same part of the brain that makes the decision and compels us to action, then what stops us from doing things? Lack of motivation, apathy, fear, perhaps?

End of the scientific stuff

In 1519, Hernán Cortés coined the phrase 'burn the boats' with some 600 Spaniards, 16 or so horses and 11 ships. They had landed on a vast inland plateau called Mexico. When Cortés gave the order to burn all the boats, there was no turning back, and they could only succeed or die. This was the ultimate motivation because Cortés and his men were vastly outnumbered, and there wasn't a retreat or surrender strategy in place to save their lives.

Remarkably though, the command to burn the boats had an opposite effect on his men because now, they were left with only 2 choices – die or ensure victory, which they did.

Adopt a 'burn the boats' attitude during the goal setting phase so that every setback just requires a workaround. Maintain your course with the same desire and mental resilience that was felt when the goal was first conceived.

Chart the course of action, estimate the potential pitfalls and once arriving at the plateau of action, burn the boats! Commit to it 100% and give it everything. Remember that failure only happens when we give up!

What we will cover in this chapter:

- Set goals like a boss! Write down your dreams and aspirations or create a collage of the lifestyle that you desire. Remember to include some positive statements on flip cards and read them every day.

- Most self-help books, talk about resilience as if it is a series of actions that you just do! We will give you a step by step guide that shows you HOW to acquire and build resilience that will improve every aspect of your life.

Let's examine a New Year's resolution for a second, where most of us at some point have proudly announced to the world that we will eat less, drink less alcohol and do more exercise. So since the decision has been made with a real sense of conviction, why do so many fail?
What is it in our executive decision-making process that is flawed and dooms most of us to failure within the first couple of weeks?

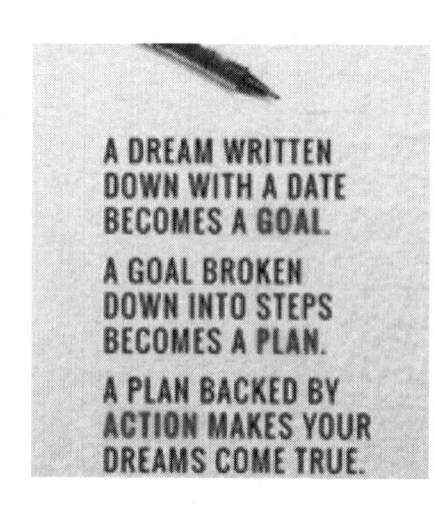

> A DREAM WRITTEN DOWN WITH A DATE BECOMES A GOAL.
>
> A GOAL BROKEN DOWN INTO STEPS BECOMES A PLAN.
>
> A PLAN BACKED BY ACTION MAKES YOUR DREAMS COME TRUE.

It has been widely speculated that as humans we try to do too much all at once, and too much change is just too much for us to handle; therefore, we give up.

Actually, it is much simpler than that, and we call this phenomenon 'overwhelm' because when we attempt to take on too much all at once, we can get that feeling of being overwhelmed. Have you ever been to a seminar or lecture, and the speaker has bombarded you with so much data that your brain wanted to pop? It's a similar principle.

There is so much information about what to eat, drink and how to exercise and, depending on what month it is, everybody can give you a different story. It's all based on someone else's opinions, and all the scientific research in the world can be shaped to fit their argument.

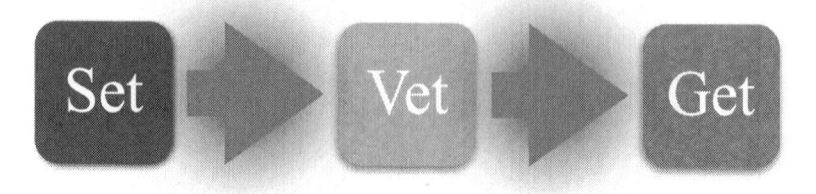

Set ➡ **Vet** ➡ **Get**

Once we have SET our heart and mind on our desired goal and before we jump in with both feet, we will need to VET it first. Choose 3-4 people that you really trust to give you some brutally honest feedback before embarking on your quest. Those people that would have no hesitation in saying that you shouldn't wear that dress because it doesn't flatter your tush.

Go and find someone that lives the life that you want to live and ask them questions so that you can get as much information about your dream as possible. One of my clients had always wanted a Porsche 911 since he was a little boy, and it had always been a pipe dream for him as he believed that he couldn't afford one.

Taking my advice, he went out to the Porsche garage and booked himself a test drive. The garage had pulled out all the stops and let him have the top of the range £127k car for the day. He was so excited, and even though he was initially unsure where he could get the money to buy one, he was reassured when I told him that the money wasn't important in this exercise.

The next day we spoke on the phone, he said, 'I'm so glad that I took your advice and test drove the car because I realised that I didn't like it,' and so over the next few months he test-drove some very prestigious cars and ticked them off his list.

That was until he found the car that he was desperate to own, a Maserati Quattroporte, and at the time, they were doing corporate finance deals. This meant that he could afford the car of his dreams! Now each day that he drives to work, he has a smile on his face.
If he hadn't gone out and taken the Porsche for a test drive, he would have still been having that same dream that he had been having since childhood. By vetting or finding out as much information as you can about your goal, you can decide whether it is achievable or not.

Top tip: Go and VET your dreams now!
Before we can go and GET our dreams, we need to prepare our mind, even if they are made with the right intention.

Focusing on HOW this preparation can happen – so that the mind can act upon any executive decisions that you have made – requires the mind to have conceived how it will achieve that goal. Here are a few tips:

- Start with the end in mind and work your way backwards in sequential steps until you arrive at the point of the things that you can do right now (Steven Covey, author of 7 Habits of Highly Effective People).
- Create a daily agenda and act upon each small incremental step towards your goal (Darren Hardy, author of The Compound Effect).
- Work out if the price is worth paying because, as with everything, there will be a price to pay either by your own time and energy, impact on your family or in pound notes (John Maxwell, author of Developing the Leader Within).
- 7-21 days before doing something new, like going to the gym or starting a new mid-term paper, detox and focus your mind on preparation (Caroline Leaf, author of Switch On Your Brain).

Most of our customers know that we at LBP (Lean Body Project) live, breathe and eat this stuff every day because we are aware that it only works!

The next time that you make your mind up to do something such as learn a new language or run a half marathon, turn the interference down first and prepare the mind for the intensity of change that you will have to endure to complete it.

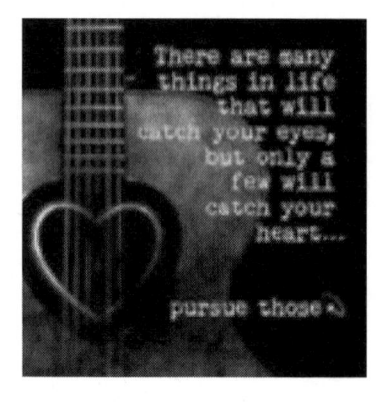

> There are many things in life that will catch your eyes, but only a few will catch your heart... pursue those

Remember this, for you to make a lifestyle choice, if the goal is audacious enough and you are really serious!

Once you have a plan of action, you just need to keep on putting one foot in front of the other and create a movement. Providing you are pointing in the right direction and moving, then you are making steady progress towards your goal no matter how small or insignificant it may seem.

We briefly mentioned resilience, which is referred a lot, especially in this day and age. The media reports that young adults need to have more of it and that is an essential ingredient in the recipe for a healthier life. It's great that we can say WHAT you need, but no one is rushing to tell you HOW to acquire it.

Here is a step-by-step guide to HOW you can become more resilient:

1. Accept that there will need to be a change. Either a change in you and your thinking and/or in your environment.
2. Continuously invest in your own development and remember in the previous chapter we said, 'who do you need to become to attain your dreams?' Where can you meet like-minded people, learn the necessary skills, and develop a greater understanding that will better prepare you for the change that is needed?
3. Take ownership of all your choices and accept the consequences of your decisions so that you can learn from any mistakes. Take charge of your own destiny, career, family and become the main character in your movie.
4. Make your purpose to continuously strive towards your goal with each of the choices that you make on a daily basis. This will help you to maintain your momentum and focus your energy when minor setbacks occur. Remember that you either find an excuse or find a way.
5. A positive shift in your thinking goes a long way because if you believe in your ability, you can adopt a can-do attitude as a result of your thinking. Then you

are more likely to have faith that your dreams are obtainable through persistence and hard work.
6. Spend some time thinking and allow your imagination to run riot, let your mind wander through the fields of your imagination. Imagine how it might feel when you obtain your dreams, what people might say about you and, in your mind's eye, how you might look. Adopt new perspectives on your journey that is sure to be filled with compromise and self-scrutiny.
7. Build relationships and invest time into them in every part of your life. This way you will be surrounded by all the resources that you might ever need, and if you find yourself giving back to that network, then it will demonstrate just how far you have come.
8. Stay true to yourself and protect your identity because with it comes integrity. It is so easy to lose part of your identity when you are trying to 'fit in' to a new environment.

Flip cards

If you, like me, need a shot of daily inspiration, each and every day to help motivate you and keep you on track, I strongly suggest that you grab yourself some index cards or coloured cards that you are able to write on.

The next stage is to write down your goals on the card but be really specific about them and be careful to use positive language and write them in the PAST TENSE. For example:

> I FEEL AMAZING NOW THAT I HAVE LOST A STONE IN WEIGHT AND ACHIEVED THE BODY SHAPE THAT I HAD ALWAYS WANTED, MY CONFIDENCE IS NOW THROUGH THE ROOF

Sounds strange at first, but there is a method behind the madness, I promise. You see, when you write down your dream, it somehow manifests into a goal. By stating what your goal is specifically and in a positive way, you are semantically priming your brain to accept what you need to do to achieve it.

Using the past tense surpasses the 'yeah right' filter in your brain, and instead, you get the 'I can do this'. Let me explain.

Your brain cannot tell the difference between what is real and what is regularly imagined. For example, if you have ever watched a horror movie and felt your heart rate increase, you know what I mean. You know that it is just a film and yet you still have a real response to what is happening on screen. This is because we empathise with the characters in the movie, which is a very human thing to do.

So by writing your goal in the past tense, it fools the mind into believing that it is attainable, regardless of what that goal might be.

If you start with one particular goal, write it on several cards and place them all over the house. I mean on the bedroom mirror, on the bathroom mirror, on the fridge door, in the car and everywhere so that you can read it daily. The next phase is to place a gold star on each and every one of your cards.

Now put more stars on your mobile, in your purse/wallet, on your credit/debit cards, photo frames, on your rear view mirror or the sun visor in the car. So that every time that you see a gold star, it will remind you of your goal and those flip cards that you have placed everywhere.

Top tip: Once you have achieved your goal, rip up the cards and start again with a new dream.

As you become more proficient with this method of goal setting, you can add in a few more goals regarding your wealth, family development, charity, spirituality or material things that you want.

My wife and I set 30 goals each year, which sounds like a lot at first, but if you consider that we take 4-5 goals relating to health, wealth, learning, giving, career, family, etc., it suddenly becomes less daunting.

Each year, between Christmas and the New Year, we sit down and review the cards that we wrote for that year and assess how we did with them. We rewrite the ones that we didn't achieve and include them in the flip cards for the following year.

What has been astounding is that each year we have surprised ourselves because we have managed to achieve 90% of our yearly goals. Now I know that it is not 100% but I don't consider 9/10 a failure either. In fact, we raise a glass of bubbly after each goal writing session and celebrate our achievements. It's now our New Year revolution!

Join us on our FB community, receive some inspiration from those taking the journey that you are about to embark upon and share your aspirations. We'd love to hear about them.

Summary

- Remember that the same part of the brain that makes the decision to get healthy is the same part of your brain that springs you to action. Delete the interference and remove the emotions from your daily decisions by planning ahead.

- Adopt a 'burn the boats' attitude and give it everything you've got as though your life depends on it because one day it just might. Show up each and every day to be the best version of you that you can possibly be.

- SET your sights on your goal and be clear why you want it so much, remembering that not everything has plausible logic behind the desire. VET your goals by testing with friends that you trust, find out as much as you can about your goal – do the research. Then you are ready to go and GET your goals, only after you have prepared your mind and accepted the changes that must happen first.

- Flip Cards. Write your cards using emotive and positive language, being specific with your words to clearly define what it is that you want. Write them all in the past tense, so your brain will accept the inevitable changes, and place them in prominent places around your environment. Oh, and the gold stars.

Workbook

- Every morning, commit to writing a gratitude statement. This is a different daily post of the things that you are grateful for AND, more importantly, give the reasons why.

- Keep a record of what you eat and drink throughout the day.

- Take a post workout selfie after each workout.

- 10 minutes daily self-development – read a book, listen to an audiobook, watch a video clip on TED, YouTube, etc.

- Ensure that you complete the daily tasks consistently for 30 days, and that INCLUDES WEEKENDS.

- Plan and record 3 goals that you want to achieve during this program.

This will be based on the fundamental principles of the 'compound effect' by Darren Hardy. This means that you build on daily choices and you will be expected to make a seemingly small change each and every day for 30 days.

After each small change, you will need to maintain that change, e.g. no caffeine for the remainder of the 30 days, and build on it ever so slightly each day. So this means that the next day:

Listen to the audiobook 'Think and grow rich' as much of it as possible: https://youtu.be/AL8NzjAkBKM

Pay particular attention to the chapter regarding DESIRE because this will help you significantly. In fact, I would go as far as to strongly suggest that you should revisit that particular chapter each day for 30 days.

Day 2 - Task 2

What are you grateful for today

Task 2 - Find a photo that shows the SHAPE that you aspire to be, it may be from yesteryear. It could simply be a photo of you when you were at you happiest! It could be simply a cut out of a magazine. Place copies of the photo around the house i.e. on the fridge, next to your bed, on your desktop, dashboard of the car etc.

I really want you to focus on the things that you WANT rather than the things that you don't!

What will I be eating today?	
Breakfast	
Lunch	
Dinner	
Snacks	

Day 3 - Task 3

What are you grateful for today

- Whenever you hear someone say that they CAN'T do something today, I want you - extraordinary people to 're-frame' what they have just said. I want you to challenge them AND/OR yourself and ask them/yourself the following question:

"What is stopping them/you?" and report some of the examples that happen around you that you have recognised.

What will I be eating today?	
Breakfast	
Lunch	
Dinner	
Snacks	

Day 4 - Task 4

What are you grateful for today

Is to get a piece of card or paper and write the goal that you have set for yourself at the end of this program. There are 3 twists:

1) you must write down with emotion
2) You must write it in the past tense
3) You must read it once a day every day for the rest of the 30 days

e.g. "I feel so happy and proud of myself now that I have the shape that I have worked so hard to get"

By writing your goal down in the *past tense* fools your subconscious mind in to believing that your goal has already happened. Now if it has already happened then it must be achievable!

What will I be eating today?	
Breakfast	
Lunch	
Dinner	
Snacks	

Day 5 - Task 5

What are you grateful for today

You know the challenges that you are going to face over the weekend already don't you?

Write down all the challenges that you KNOW that you are going to face and how you will over come them.

* The simple rule is write it in the past tense as though you have written it on Monday morning.

That way when you read it on Monday, it will be a positive start

What will I be eating today?	
Breakfast	
Lunch	
Dinner	
Snacks	

Day 6 - Task 6

What are you grateful for today

---

* Plan a menu for all of your evening meals this coming week and post it in the group and place a copy of it in your kitchen, on the fridge or above the cooker.
* Write out a shopping list full of the ingredients that you will need in order to make those meals.

This way, when you go shopping you will know exactly what you NEED to buy rather than what you WANT to buy.

Use the template provided in the appendix

What will I be eating today?	
Breakfast	
Lunch	
Dinner	
Snacks	

Day 7 - Task 7

What are you grateful for today

Your task is to use positive words when talking to yourself, describing yourself or talking to others especially after a workout! focus on the positive effects of you training, so maybe you're feeling energised, proud of yourself or feeling toned!

Make a not of the positive statements about yourself or any compliments that you may have received from Friends, family or work colleagues.

Find a genuine reason to pay someone a compliment today and make their day.

What will I be eating today?	
Breakfast	
Lunch	
Dinner	
Snacks	

Day 8 - Task 8

What are you grateful for today

Identify something about yourself that you don't like and that you would like to change or forget and lose forever. e.g. impatience, I want instant results and I want them now. Then imagine that you are sat in a window seat of a carriage, on a train at your local train station about to travel to your favourite destination. On the platform is your dopple ganger (your identical twin) and they are demonstrating the very characteristic that you don't like about yourself. Now here is the secret to this. As the train pulls away, you keep looking back at the platform and you notice that your dopple ganger becomes smaller and smaller until you pull away in to the distance and the platform is just a speck in the distance.

What will I be eating today?	
Breakfast	
Lunch	
Dinner	
Snacks	

Day 9 - Task 9

What are you grateful for today

Introducing 'Parkinson's' time law "work expands to fill the time that it is allotted"

This means that whatever time we allow to complete a task, we will generally do it in that said time. This usually works by leaving it until the last minute and then working twice as hard to complete it!

Plan out your day from the time that you wake in the morning to the time that you go to bed. Tell me where you can improve and be more efficient with your time. Write down the improvements that you will make.

What will I be eating today?	
Breakfast	
Lunch	
Dinner	
Snacks	

Day 10 - Task 10

What are you grateful for today

Building on yesterday's task where I'm sure that you have suggested some excellent ways to improve and be more efficient.

Today is about your daily agenda and the 'story' that you tell yourself everyday! Either your inner child buy's your story OR your inner child buy's YOUR story AND it's your choice.

Then you can either examine it yourself or ask someone else to do it for you. Is it a genuine story or is it just an excuse?

Recognise the stories that you tell yourself and write them down and label them either TRUE or FALSE

What will I be eating today?	
Breakfast	
Lunch	
Dinner	
Snacks	

Day 11 - Task 11

What are you grateful for today

Simple task today, answer this question and write it on a post it note and pin it some where prominent:

What one thing will you differently today that will help you achieve your goal, that you haven't done so far in the last 13 days?

What will I be eating today?	
Breakfast	
Lunch	
Dinner	
Snacks	

Day 12 - Task 12

To prepare you for the 2nd weekend, we thought that we would give you a checklist to help you stay on track:

1) Are you readying all your food for the weekend OR just the working week? Remember that you still need to eat on Saturday and Sunday.
2) Are you drinking enough water? If your body is dehydrated, then it will retain water, which in turn will make you feel bloated.
3) Are you getting enough protein? Remember that your body will repair itself quicker and burn fat better if you eat your recommended amount of protein.
4) Are you consuming too many liquid calories, including alcohol, fizzy drinks, fruit juices, etc.?
5) Are you getting enough sleep? What time do you plan to go to bed? Research shows that a good night's sleep is essential to weight loss.
6) Do you consistently eat breakfast? It should be one of those meals that are pre-prepared and planned in.
7) Do you shop with a specific list in mind or do you still shop daily depending on what you FANCY to eat that night?
8) Keeping a food diary of all that you eat and drink (even on a night out) can help you balance out some of your other choices over the weekend.
9) Consistency is a major factor in your results so breaking the healthy routine over the weekend (especially with alcohol) means that by the time it's out of your system (72 hours), it'll be Wednesday before your body begins to burn fat again.
10) Remember to stay the course, you've come this far. As long as you keep putting one foot in front of the other, you will eventually get there. Keep moving forward.

Now on the next page, you will find a list of numbers from 1-10. Your task is to rate yourself on a scale of 1-10 on how well you are doing with each of the statements above.

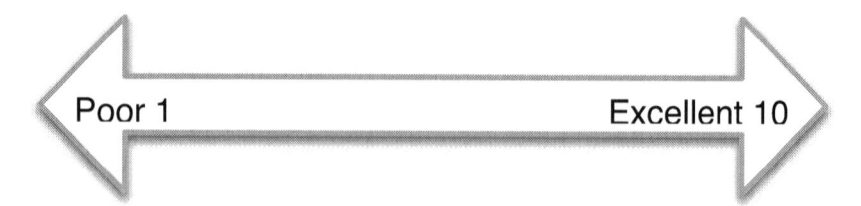

Poor 1 ⟷ Excellent 10

Day 12 - Task 12 continued

WHAT ARE YOU GRATEFUL FOR TODAY

Your mission today is to check off the list those that you have nailed and have well under control.

1)
2)
3)
4)
5)
6)
7)
8)
9)
10)

What will I be eating today?

Breakfast	
Lunch	
Dinner	
Snacks	

Day 13 - Task 13

What are you grateful for today

Your task today is to post photo's of your pre prepared meals in the LBP Facebook community - Thats it.

That is assuming that you have preprepared your meals today for the whole week.

What we do normally is put them in to plastic cartons with lids and then freeze them. Take out what you need the night before to give them time to defrost.

What will I be eating today?	
Breakfast	
Lunch	
Dinner	
Snacks	

Day 14 - Task 14

It's the weekend again, and it's one of my favourite times because it means I get a lay in, a leisurely walk with the dog and later the family gets together for a meal.

It's also a good day to make yourself ready for the week, so here is a little something to help you. **PLAN AHEAD.**

PREDETERMINE a course of action set goals.
PREPARATION is the key and PASSION is the driving force to get you there and professionalism to maintain the discipline of your choices.
LAY out your plan starting with the end in mind and work backwards.
ADJUST your priorities so that everything you do contributes towards that goal especially for the next 19 days.
NOTIFY key people in your life and ask for their support. Even more important, tell them 'HOW' you want them to help you, e.g. your drinking buddies.

ALLOW time for acceptance in your mind. Merely making a decision is different to acting upon that decision. Prepare your mind first!
HEAD into action and give it everything that you have got and leave nothing in the tank. Remove the emotion from the decision process, and you will succeed.
EXPECT challenges and welcome them as an opportunity to demonstrate your resilience and determination 'bring it on'.
ALWAYS point to the successes and learn from everything else. This way, you will always succeed!
DAILY review of your plan will help you navigate through the naysayers and stop life getting in your way. At the end of each day, before you close your eyes, ask yourself, 'Did I do what I wanted today?'

Day 14 - Task 14 continued

What are you grateful for today

What were the major challenges that you faced over the weekend that are stopping you from getting the results that you want? For those of you that are still facing the same barriers, It is time to be honest with yourselves! What story are you telling yourself because it is time to 'wake up and smell the coffee'

Post 3 goals that you are going to achieve in the next 7 days (this includes the weekend)
Goal 1 I am going to........
Goal 2 I am going to........
Goal 3 I am going to........

What will I be eating today?	
Breakfast	
Lunch	
Dinner	
Snacks	

Day 15 - Task 15

What are you grateful for today

Think of a forfeit for yourself for failing to achieve the goals that you have already committed to. If you're brave enough to involve your family or friends, I'm sure that they'll have a few suggestions for you.

There is a twist though - you can allocate the forfeit to someone else in your network of friends or family on a first come first served basis if you achieve all of YOUR goals.

You could donate to children's charity, do someone else's stair climbs, take the neighbours trash out or simply pay for a night out.

What will I be eating today?	
Breakfast	
Lunch	
Dinner	
Snacks	

Day 16 - Task 16

What are you grateful for today

What do you want people to say about you? What would be your mission statement?

E.g. "I want to be loved by some, liked by many but respected by all"

In addition, how does this help you achieve your goal?

E.g. "Set an example to those closest to me, add value to everyone that I meet on a daily basis and by living a breathing everything that I preach"

Write down your mission statement & how it will help you achieve your goals.

What will I be eating today?	
Breakfast	
Lunch	
Dinner	
Snacks	

Day 17 - Task 17

What are you grateful for today

What ever it is that you desire in life, the price is the price. You can't haggle with destiny and get what you want for a bargain or negotiate a discount!

If it takes 60 days to achieve the shape that you want, then it takes 60 consecutive days of dedication and sacrifices. It isn't 44 days sacrifice (accounting for weekends) and 16 days half hearted, the price is 60 consecutive days.

Over the remaining 12 days, what sacrifices do you anticipate needing to make in order to move closer to your dream?

What will I be eating today?

Breakfast	
Lunch	
Dinner	
Snacks	

Day 18 - Task 18

What are you grateful for today

How serious are you about achieving your goal on a scale of 1-10? 1 being not very serious at all, to 10 being that it completely consumes your daily thoughts.

Post your score and then answer the following questions

3 questions:
1) What have you done to move you away from your goal?
2) What have you done to move you towards your goal?
3) What steps will you NOW take?

What will I be eating today?	
Breakfast	
Lunch	
Dinner	
Snacks	

Day 19 - Task 19

What are you grateful for today

Scenario a: do you inform your friends that you need their support and that if they continue to lead you astray.

Scenario b: tolerate their influence and laugh it off, knowing that you are sabotaging your future happiness

Scenario c: are you able to remain determined and get your own drink from the bar because your friends wont order you a lime and soda

What are you currently tolerating in your life right now that is taking you away from your goals?

What will I be eating today?	
Breakfast	
Lunch	
Dinner	
Snacks	

Day 20 - Task 20

What are you grateful for today

List all the things that make you happy and then identify the feeling you get when they happen and write them down. What do you need to get in order to be happy?

What is your happiness model?

It could be a lazy Sunday, going for a long stroll withe dog, spending time with your spouse, watching sport, exercising or family meals.

Then make sure that you do at least one of those everyday.

What will I be eating today?

Breakfast	
Lunch	
Dinner	
Snacks	

Day 21 - Task 21

What are you grateful for today

If you have succeeded in your goals then congratulations and you should post 3 more goals even bigger than last week that you will achieve in the last 8 days of this program. Plus post in the group the words to describe how you are feeling especially on a Monday.

If you failed in your tasks this week, then apart from you forfeit, you need to listen to the story that you are telling yourself and be honest with yourself as to why you failed this week.

Either way what have you learned from the experiences this week?

What will I be eating today?	
Breakfast	
Lunch	
Dinner	
Snacks	

Day 22 - Task 22

What are you grateful for today

Be honest with yourselves and kind to yourselves at the same time. I know that this might seem like an oxymoron but stay with me.

Being kind to yourself is looking in the mirror and noticing all the things that you LIKE about yourself (body included - there must be something) and notice the thing that you would most like to change about body too.

Provide examples of 1 thing you LIKE about your body and 1 thing that you would most like to IMPROVE and how many of the 84600 seconds a day will you invest in doing so?

What will I be eating today?	
Breakfast	
Lunch	
Dinner	
Snacks	

Day 23 - Task 23

What are you grateful for today

First of all give your inner child a name that is different to yours, imagine what he/she looks like, how they might sound and how you feel when they resent themselves.

* Recognising the emotional feelings that you are having and the situation that you are in and then I want you to imagine that it is your inner child dropping to the floor kicking and screaming like a toddler that can't have its own way.

Make a note of your experiences and if you are still finding this a challenge, stay strong and join our online community on Facebook

What will I be eating today?	
Breakfast	
Lunch	
Dinner	
Snacks	

Day 24 - Task 24

What are you grateful for today

_____

Be deliberate with the amount of time that you devote to charity or giving back to society.

Being inspired with a random act of kindness I thought that I would encourage you to do something kind for a complete stranger, without expecting anything in return and see how you feel afterwards.

E.g. pay for the coffee of the person behind you in the cue in the cafe and Tweet or Facebook message a genuine compliment to three people right now.

What will I be eating today?	
Breakfast	
Lunch	
Dinner	
Snacks	

Day 25 - Task 25

What are you grateful for today

Now for some real goal setting! Not the mamby pamby ones that those company courses tell you about. You know - the SMART ones etc. I mean the Big Hairy Audacious Goal (BHAG)

What has been the thing that you have always wanted to do?

It might be travelling around the world, writing a book, become an actress, play a musical instrument or learn a new language.

What ever it is that has been eating away in side you write it down and put a deadline on it and place it some where prominent.

What will I be eating today?	
Breakfast	
Lunch	
Dinner	
Snacks	

Day 26 - Task 26

What are you grateful for today

Take the time to tag someone you are connected to on social media and post something really positive and sincere about them.

Make it specific, relevant and remember to include the reason why in your post:

E.g. "Damien Coates has been inspirational over the past 30 days because he has managed to maintain his activity, deal with challenges in his personal life and still managed to find time to train most mornings"

What will I be eating today?	
Breakfast	
Lunch	
Dinner	
Snacks	

Day 27 - Task 27

What are you grateful for today

What's your sentence?

Your sentence is something that you want people to say about you in your absence. So it may be as simple as:

"She inspired others to complete Rough Runner for a good cause and got everyone across the finish line"

Simply write your sentence or write what you think someone else's sentence should be and tell them, remember to explain why.

What will I be eating today?	
Breakfast	
Lunch	
Dinner	
Snacks	

Day 28 - Task 28

What are you grateful for today

When I look back at my life and remember the people that I have met, the jobs that I have had and the destinations that I have travelled to, I feel extremely fortunate.

Post the top 10 things have you achieved in your life.

It could be that you got a 1st class honours degree or that you completed a total warrior or simply be having your children.

What will I be eating today?	
Breakfast	
Lunch	
Dinner	
Snacks	

Day 29 - Task 29

What are you grateful for today

It's the penultimate day in the 30 day program and as always I have something special lined up for you.

There is a phrase that is used so much in life and that is "In hind sight"

If you could travel back in time to 30 days ago and give yourself some advice, what would that advice be?

Start your post as follows: A note to my younger self "..............."

What will I be eating today?	
Breakfast	
Lunch	
Dinner	
Snacks	

Day 30 - Task 30

What are you grateful for today

Looking back over the past 30 days what has stood out the most for you?

What mind tool has made the biggest difference for you?

Have any one of you had any epiphanies and if so when was the turning point?

Having completed the 30 days could you have gone on for longer if so how long?

What will I be eating today?	
Breakfast	
Lunch	
Dinner	
Snacks	

Congratulations on completing the 30-day program! We sincerely hope that you have enjoyed it and taken lots of things from it.

You NOW have a choice to make: YOU can either continue to develop yourselves through this path you have already been travelling for 30 days OR go back to how you were and what feels comfortable.

The fact is that the change doesn't have to be difficult, BUT because we don't like it, we make it difficult for ourselves. The world is constantly changing and evolving and so must we if we want to stay ahead and be successful in life.

What now? Have you got the staying power to complete our 90-day online program? If you have, then you can request our special VIP discount via the email below.

We do have several options for you. If you have joined our FB community, then you also have access to our VIP lounge. This is where we continually provide the latest healthy recipes, exercises, coaching and support to keep you on your journey.

We, at LBP, would like to hear from you with your thoughts or questions, and we are almost always available through social media. We are on a mission to help one million people to choose a healthier life and achieve the body shape that will make them happy.

We want to start a movement by educating people that have been misled by false advertising so that we can live longer and reduce the strain on our NHS system.

Most of the common diseases that plague this century can be at a cellular level caused by what we eat, drink and how we live our lives.

Thank you for taking the time to read this book, and if you have enjoyed it, you can tell others about it. That way, you can help someone else who may be in the same position as you and will benefit from the book as well. But if you didn't, please contact us at info@theleanbodyproject.co.uk. We would love to hear your thoughts.

In conclusion to my story from the beginning of this book, I have taken a 12-month journey from being out of shape to having the kind of body that I can be proud of on a beach.

I'm not saying that it was easy and that I didn't have weekends where I overindulged with food and alcohol because I definitely did. The difference is that they were just a few days and then I slipped back into the healthy regime immediately.

If I had any advice for anyone that is thinking of getting in shape, it would be this: 'Prepare your mind before you embark on the journey.'

My wife has picked up the gauntlet and joined me on this voyage. She consistently makes clean food for us to eat and she prepares her food like a boss!

The support of the LBP community is a contributing factor to her sticking to the strategy. I have to give her credit because since she has been well enough to get up and move, she has made plane to join in regular exercises classes and the proof is definitely in the pudding.

Maybe we will write a sequel that depicts her journey. It's for real people that have to juggle their lives around kids, school, work, running a home and social gatherings. Life has a way of getting in the way of a perfectly laid plan, and somehow you need to navigate through it to succeed.

I cannot stress enough the power of positivity through those prolonged and painful periods, where I could quite easily have given up. It has helped me through the most stressful times when I had been scratching around for money trying to get my business off the ground. All the times where prayer had been the saviour of my sanity on many occasions.

Through every difficult period in your life, whether you have been insulted because of your weight or told that you were ugly or that you weren't worth anything. To those of you that have mental scars from your childhood that run so deep that they make you feel empty or have tried every diet and exercise under the sky and still have failed to stick to it for more than a few weeks and to those of you that lack confidence and self-esteem, I say, 'you are enough,' you make a difference to the world. I believe in each and every one of you!

'We, ourselves, feel that what we are doing is just a drop in the ocean. But the ocean would be less because of that missing drop.' ~ Mother Teresa

It is our sincere wish for you is that you can improve your life even by one degree as a direct result of reading this book then we will consider that a success.

The LBP team is on a mission to help one million people make better choices when it comes to their health, to improve and enrich their lives by providing them with the continued support so that they can achieve the dreams and have the lives that they really deserve.

So, as part of our gift to you for buying this book, you can have access to the 3-month online program for only £49.99!

The normal retail price for this is £199.99 plus vat, which means that you are making a huge **saving of 75%!**

Incredible? And I'm sure you will love the program, especially if you enjoyed completing this one.

As a special offer, we will give you exclusive access to our **prestige package**, which includes daily workouts, healthy menus and cooking videos.

If that isn't enough, there is more! This unbelievable package will also give you access to our **VIP area**; that means daily shots of motivation, plus hints and tips from our professional PTs and mindset coaches.

We will be doing **webinars** for you to watch at your leisure and **live Q & A** for you to post your questions in advance, where we will do our very best to answer them as honestly as possible.

You will be able to book your places on our **MOM** (Mind Over Mass) **workshops** either through the website, the VIP group on Facebook or contact us on infor@theleanbodyproject.co.uk

Follow my progress of Facebook and see what I have managed to achieved in just 8 weeks! I can obtain a very flat stomach and demonstrate great abs but, alas, it is not natural or healthy to be that shredded all the time.

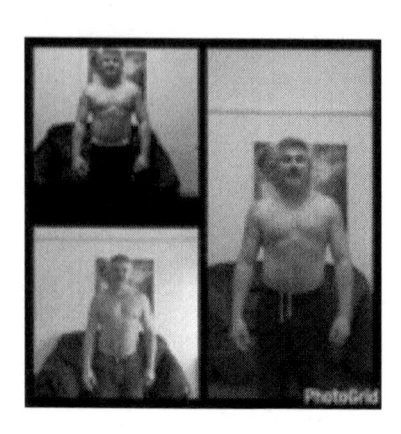

I could have quite easily posted my photos with a six-pack digitally enhanced torso, just to sell my book, but that would have been incongruent, and I want to maintain my authenticity and integrity.

I will keep going until I can post a six pack but I am at least another 7 weeks diet and hard work away from that just yet. If you would like to keep up to date with my progress, then please join us on Facebook or one of our next seminars!

Our sincere wish is for you to be happy and live the life that you desire!

Having just returned from a much needed holiday in Italy. I am happy to say that I haven't gained much in the way of weight and although I thoroughly enjoyed my holiday and relaxed. I still made some choices that limited the damage of indulgence.

The truth of the matter is that it is un-natural for us as humans to be so lean and obtaining a six pack will take approximately 16 weeks.

A healthy fat % to muscle ratio is said to be somewhere between 14-18% in men unless you are wanting to compete

In conclusion - whatever your goal is you also need to live and enjoy your life to the fullest. Remember that daily compromise, consistency and choices are the key elements to your success.

References and further reading:

The Compound Effect - Darren Hardy

Good to Great - Jim Collins

Miracle Morning - Hal Elrod

You Can Be Thin - Marissa Peers

The Slight Edge - Jeff Olson

Today Matters - John C Maxwell

15 Invaluable Laws of Growth - John C Maxwell

Get Control of Sugar - Paul McKenna

Office for National Statistics - www.ons.gov.uk

Sleep The Unsung Hero of Fat Loss - www.bodybuilding.com, science daily.com, www.womenshealthmag.com, www.mensfitness.com, sleepfoundation.org, Sleep.org

Lean Body Solution - Damien Coates

The Ultimate Body Transformation Plan - Nick Mitchell

Upgrade Your Life - Pat Divilly

Sane - Emma Young

Getting Things Done - David Allen

Crazy Sexy Diet - Kris Carr

Introducing NLP - O'Connor and Seymour

- Flipnosis - Kevin Dutton
- Thinking Fast and Slow - Daniel Kahneman
- Chicken Soup for The Soul - Lack Canfield et al.
- The Pursuit of Happiness - Chris Gardner
- 59 Seconds - Richard Wiseman
- Rhinoceros Success - Scott Alexander
- The Cortisol Connection - Shawn Talbot
- Make Your Life Great - Richard Bandler
- Think and Grow Rich - Napoleon Hill
- 7 Habits of Highly Successful People - Steven Covey
- The Science of Behaviour - Carlson et al.
- Into The Silent Land - Paul Broks
- More Than a Game - Phil Jackson
- Dare to Dream - John Ryan
- Winning - Clive Woodward
- Fitness Motivation - Rejeski and Kenny
- Guerrilla Coaching - Glen McCoy
- Blink - Malcolm Gladwell
- Drive - Daniel Pink
- A Whole New Mind - Daniel Pink
- Mind Over Fatter - Anna Richardson
- Daring Greatly - Brene Brown

Burn The Fat Feed the Muscle - Tom Venuto

Start with Why - Simon Sinek

Appendix

Here are some night time affirmations for you:

I have had a productive day and I am content

I am now ready to go to sleep

My body is relaxed and my mind is quiet

I am grateful for the roof over my head and this bed that I sleep in

I am lucky to have people in my life that care about me

Tomorrow I will wake up feeling refreshed and full of energy

I feel at peace right now as I lay my head down on my pillow

I remember all the good that I have done today

I will make somebodies day tomorrow

I am falling asleep with only good positive thoughts in my mind

I will be grateful when I awake in the morning

I am really sleepy now and my mind is quiet

Meal Planner and shopping list template

Monday	
Tuesday	
Wednesday	
Thursday	
Friday	
Saturday	
Sunday	

Shopping list:

Keep a record of what exercises you complete &/or
Plan out your exercise routines in advance

Exercise	Reps	Sets	Weight

Printed in Great Britain
by Amazon